ORGANON OF THE ART OF HEALING

ORGANON OF THE ART OF HEALING

By

SAMUEL HAHNEMANN,

FIFTH AMERICAN EDITION

TRANSLATED FROM THE FIFTH GERMAN EDITION,

BY

C. WESSELHOEFT, M.D.

GYAN

Published by

Gyan Publishing House
5, Ansari Road
Daryaganj, New Delhi-110002
Phone: 011-47034999, 9811692060
E-mail: books@gyanbooks.com

Distribution Network
gyanbooks.com
India, USA, Canada, UK, Australia, France

ISBN : 978-81-212-6699-4 (PB)
First Published, 1876

2nd Impression 2022

Printed at: Gyan Press, Delhi.

ORGANON OF THE ART OF HEALING
Author: SAMUEL HAHNEMANN

ORGANON

OF

BY

SAMUEL HAHNEMANN.

AUDE SAPERE.

FIFTH AMERICAN EDITION,

TRANSLATED FROM THE FIFTH GERMAN EDITION,

BY

C. WESSELHOEFT, M.D.

1876.

CONTENTS.

INTRODUCTION.

A REVIEW OF "PHYSIC" AS HITHERTO PRACTICED, ALLOPATHY, AND PALLIATIVE CURE OF THE OLD SCHOOL OF MEDICINE.

SINCE man existed he has singly or in numbers been exposed to diseases derived from physical or moral causes. During his primitive state of nature, man needed but few remedies, since a simple mode of living admitted but few diseases; together with the development of the human race into communities, the causes of diseases, and the necessity for methods of cure increased with even pace. From that time forward (soon after Hippocrates, that is, since two and a half thousand years), the treatment of rapidly and variously increasing diseases became the occupation of men, who conceitedly endeavored to invent modes of relief by processes of reason and conjecture. A countless variety of opinions on the nature of diseases and their remedies, sprang from a great variety of minds, and the theoretical products of their fancies were called (structures) *systems*, each contradicting the others as well as itself. At first these sophistical representations stupefied the reader into astonishment at their unintelligible wisdom, and drew around the originator of the system a host of imitators of this unnatural sophistry. These disciples, however, had little time or success in practicing what they had learned, before the system, so called, was superseded by another often entirely opposite, and destined to a like transient reputation and existence. None, however, were in harmony with nature and experience; they were theoretical fabrications of astute minds, nominally drawn from principles utterly useless in practice at the bedside, on account of their subtlety and opposition to nature, and served only as subjects for empty disputations.

Independently of all these theories, there was developed at the same time a manner of cure with unknown, mixed medicinal substances, intended for gratuitously constructed forms of disease, arranged according to material ideas contradicting nature and experience, and, hence, necessarily of evil result, called "old medicine," allopathy.

Without ignoring the merits of many physicians in relation to the auxiliary sciences pertaining to medicine, such as the advancement of physics and chemistry, natural history in its different branches, and of man particularly, anthropology, physiology, anatomy, etc., I shall now only consider the practical part of medicine, that of curing, in order to show how imperfectly diseases have hitherto been treated. It is not my purpose, however, to notice that mechanical routine of dealing with precious human life according to pocket-formularies, the continued publication of which proves their still frequent use. I leave that unnoticed as the scandalous habit of the scum of vulgar practitioners. I speak only of the hitherto existing medical art, which deems itself scientific on account of its antiquity.

This ancient school of medicine boasted much of its ability to say that its practice alone deserved the name of "*rational* medicine," because it alone searched for, or sought to remove the *cause of disease, and that it proceeded in its management of diseases in imitation of nature.*

Tolle causam! is the repeated cry; but their achievements ended with that cry. *They fancied they could find the cause of disease;* but did not find it, because it is unrecognizable and not to be found. Since many, indeed, by far the greater number of diseases are of dynamic (spirit-like) origin and dynamic nature, their cause, therefore, remaining unrecognizable by our senses, it became necessary to invent a cause. For this purpose they inspected the parts of the normal, dead human body (anatomy), and compared them with the visible changes in the corresponding parts in diseased subjects (pathological anatomy). They instituted comparisons between the phenomena and functions of healthy life (physiology), and the endless deviations therefrom occurring in countless morbid conditions (pathology, semeiology). They proceeded to draw conclusions from these deviations regarding the invisible process of change going on in the inward structure of the diseased human organism, and shaped these conclusions into a fanciful picture which theoretical medicine mistook for the *prima causa morbi*;[1] also, for the proximate cause of disease, the inner nature of disease, and, in fact, *the disease itself*, forgetting the axiom of common sense, that the cause of a thing or event cannot be the thing or event itself.

How, then, was it possible, without self-deception, to make this internal, invisible essence their object of cure, and to prescribe for it medicines with curative tendencies, likewise most unknown, and above all to make use of several unknown medicines mixed together in so-called recipes?

But this sublime project of discovering *a priori* an internal, invisible cause of disease, was changed (at least in the hands of those old-school physicians of wiser conceit) into a search for that cause, however, under the guidance of symptoms; thus by conjectures they tried to determine first the general *character* of a given case of disease,[2] and then to find if it were cramp, debility, paralysis, fever, inflammation, induration, or deposits in one part or another, or plethora, insufficiency or superabundance in the juices of oxygen, carbon, hydrogen, or nitrogen; increased or depressed arterial, venous or capillary circulation; relative proportion of the factors of sensibility, irritability or reproduction. Such conjectures, honored by the hitherto existing school with the name of causal indication, and regarded as the only possible rationality in medicine, were only deceptive and hypothetical assumptions, never destined *to be either practical or useful.* They were unfit, even if they had, or could have been well founded, to indicate the most appropriate remedy in a case of disease; mere conjectures which, although flattering the self-esteem of the learned author, generally lead him astray in practice. Such were the notions designed rather for the sake of ostentation than as means of finding curative indications.

How often *e. g.*, there appeared to be cramp or paralysis in one part of the organism, while inflammation occurred in another!

Or, whence, on the other hand, could the infallible remedies for each of these alleged general characters come? The most infallible remedies could have been no less than *specifics, i. e.* medicines homogeneous[3] in their action with the morbific irritation (Krankheits-Reize). The use of these specifics, however, had been prohibited[4] and condemned, as extremely injurious by the old school; because observation had taught that such medicines, in the customary large doses, had proved to be dangerous on account of the highly increased receptivity in disease for homogeneous irritation. The old school, however, had no presentiment of minute and extremely minute doses. Cures, then, were not and could not be performed in the direct (natural) manner, by means of homogeneous, specific medicines which were, and continued to be unknown in regard to the fullest extent of their effects; and even if this knowledge had existed, such generalizing views would have made it impossible to conjecture the appropriate remedy.

But since it began, after all, to appear more reasonable to seek, if possible, another more direct path in the place of circuitous measures, the old school of medicine proceeded to cancel disease directly by eliminating the (alleged) *material cause of disease;* indeed, it was almost impossible for the common school of practitioners, in contemplating and judging a disease, or in seeking the indications for its cure, to free their minds from these ideas of materiality, or to recognize the nature of an organism both spiritual and material, as a being so highly potentiated, that the modification of its life, called disease, manifested by sensations and functions, must alone be regarded as conditioned and effected by means of dynamic (spirit-like) influences, and that such sensations and functions could be effected by no other cause.

Such morbidly altered materials, abnormal turgescences, as well as secretions, were throughout regarded by the old school as exciters, or, at least in respect to their reaction, as maintainers of disease, and they are considered as such to this day.

Therefore that school believed in the achievement of causal cures by endeavoring to eliminate those imaginary and supposed causes of disease. Hence their busy endeavors at removing bile in bilious fevers by vomiting;[5] hence their emetics in so-called gastro-ataxia,[6] and their officiousness in purging out mucus, ascarides, or lumbricoids in pallor of the countenance, voraciousness, colic, and tumid belly of children.[7] Hence their venesections in hæmorrhages,[8] and hence, principally, all sorts of bloodletting,[9] considered by that school as a chief indication in inflammations, which process they now imagine to exist in almost every morbidly affected part of the body, and the removal of which, by means of a fatal number of leeches, they consider as their duty, therein following the precedence of a well-known bloodthirsty physician of Paris (like sheep following the bellwether even into the hands of the butcher). They think, in this manner genuine causal indications are obeyed, and rational cures performed. Furthermore, by ligation of polypi, by excision of indolent glandular swellings, or by their destruction through artificial suppuration, excited by irritating local applications; by enucleation of fatty (steatomatous, melicerous) tumors; by operating upon aneurisms, lachrymal and rectal fistulæ; by excision of scirrhous breasts, amputation of necrosed limbs, etc., physicians of the old school consider that they have radically cured the patient, and have performed causal cures. They persist in this belief, when they make use of their *repellentia*, when they exsiccate inveterate, ichorous ulcers of the leg with astringent applications; with oxides of lead, copper, or zinc (perhaps making incidental use of laxatives, thereby producing debility, without relieving the fundamental disorder); when they cauterize a chancre; destroy cauliflower excrescences by local applications; dispel the itch from the surface by ointments of sulphur, oxides of lead, quicksilver, or zinc; suppress ophthalmia with solutions of lead or zinc, or when they drive rheumatic pains from the limbs by means of opodeldoc, volatile liniments, or fumigations with cinnabar or amber. In all such cases they profess to have controlled the disorder, conquered the disease, and to have executed causal cures. But mark the result! Metaschematisms (metastases), sure to appear sooner or later (but which are then pronounced as new diseases), *and invariably more serious than the primary disorder*, refute their assertions sufficiently, and could or should undeceive them by disclosing the deeper, immaterial nature of the evil, as well as its dynamic (spirit-like) origin, to be combated only by dynamic processes.

In modern times (not to say up to the present time) the common school was in the habit of presupposing the existence of morbid matter (and acrids) which, however subtle it might have been considered, they sought to remove from the blood and lymphatics by the exhalations, the perspiration, and the urinary apparatus, or through the action of the salivary glands; to eject them in the shape of sputa from the tracheal and bronchial follicles; and by making use of emetics and cathartics to clear them out of the stomach and intestines—all for the purpose of expelling the material exciting cause of the disease from the body, and thus fulfilling the conditions for a thorough causal cure.

By means of incisions into the skin of the diseased body, into which foreign substances were introduced, thereby producing chronic ulcers, fontanels, and setons continued for years, the old school endeavored to draw off the *materia peccans* from the diseased body (always affected only dynamically), as filthy fluids are drawn from a barrel through a faucet. In like manner it was attempted to remove noxious humors by perpetual application of cantharides and spurge, thus only weakening the diseased body to the verge of incurability by all these inconsiderate and unnatural procedures.

I admit that it was more convenient for human weakness to assume, in the treatment of diseases, the existence of some morbid matter, perceptible by means of the senses (particularly because the patients themselves easily inclined to such an idea), having discovered which, nothing remained to be done but to procure the requisite quantities of remedies to cleanse the blood and juices, to promote the secretion of urine and perspiration, to assist expectoration from the chest, or to scour the stomach and intestines. On this account scarcely anything is found in all works on Materia Medica, from Dioscorides to those of the present time, regarding the individual remedies, and the special, proper action of each; besides references to their supposed utility in this or that *pathological name*, remedies are alluded to only with regard to their properties as augmenting the flow of urine, perspiration, secretions of the chest, or menses; but particular stress is laid upon their power of producing an upward or downward evacuation from the alimentary canal; because the only aim and object of practical physicians has ever been the evacuation of some material morbific substance, as well as of several kinds of fictitious humors, alleged to form the basis of diseases.

But these were all vain dreams, unfounded suppositions, and hypotheses, shrewdly invented for the convenience of therapeutics, according to which diseases were most readily cured by the expulsion of material morbific matters, if such, indeed, existed!

But the essential nature of diseases and their cure, cannot accommodate themselves to such dreams, or to the convenience of physicians; diseases will not cease to be (spiritual) *dynamic aberrations of our spirit-like life, manifested by sensations and actions; that is, they will not cease, for the sake of those foolish and groundless hypotheses, to be immaterial modifications of our sensorial condition* (health).

These causes of our diseases cannot be material ones, since the least foreign material substance[10], however mild it may appear to us, if introduced into our bloodvessels, is suddenly expelled like a poison by our vital force; or, where that is impossible, death is the result. Even if the smallest splinter is by accident inserted into our sensitive parts, that vital principle, omnipresent in the interior of our body, does not rest until the offending substance has been removed by pain, fever, suppuration, or sloughing. How happens it then, for instance, in a case of eruptive disease of twenty years' standing, that this indefatigable, active vital principle should patiently tolerate in the juices for twenty years a foreign, inimical, material eruptive substance (Ausschlags-Stoff) such as herpetic, scrofulous, or gouty humors? What nosologist ever beheld with bodily eyes such morbific matter, that he should speak so confidently of it, and make it the basis of a medical procedure? Who has ever been able to prove the existence of the poison of gout or of scrofula by ocular demonstration?[11]

Even if some material substance, brought in contact with the skin or a wound, had propagated diseases by infection, who can prove (as has often been asserted in our works on pathogeny) that some material particle of that substance had mingled with, or had been absorbed by the juices of our body? Washing the sexual organs, even if immediately and carefully done, never is a protection against infection by venereal chancre. A breath of air wafted over from one afflicted by small-pox, can call forth this horrible disease in a healthy child.

How much in weight of material matter could have been absorbed in this manner by the juices, in order to produce, in the first instance, if left uncured, a painfully tormenting disease (syphilis), terminating only with the remotest period of life, that is with death, and to produce, in the second instance, a disease, rapidly fatal by its tendency to general suppuration[12] (human small-pox)?

Is it possible to admit the existence of material morbific matter and its transition into the blood in this and all such cases? A letter written in the sick-room, and sent a great distance, has often imparted to the recipient the same miasmatic disease. Can material morbific matter be thought of in this case as having permeated the humors of the body? But why all these proofs? Has not dangerous bilious fever been known to result from a mortifying altercation? Has not a superstitious prophecy of death been known to come true at the predicted time; or a sudden arrival of sad or exceedingly joyful tidings to have caused instantaneous death? Where, in such instances, is the material morbific substance said to have passed bodily over into the organism, where it is supposed to have begotten and maintained a disease, and without the actual removal and ejection of which substance a radical cure is said to be impossible?

The defenders of an assumption so gross as that of morbific matters, should blush to have so inconsiderately overlooked and misunderstood the spiritual nature of life, as well as the spiritual dynamic power of pathogenetic causes; thereby having degraded themselves to the level of medical scavengers (Fegeärzte), who, instead of curing, destroyed life by their endeavors to expel morbific matter from the diseased body, where it never existed.

Are those loathsome and impure discharges in diseases the source and maintainers of the latter, or, on the contrary, are they not always *effete products of the disease itself, that is to say, of a dynamical disturbance and modification of life?*

Considering these wrong material views concerning the origin and nature of diseases, it was no wonder, that in all ages the efforts of little and great practitioners, as well as the invention of the sublimest medical systems, were invariably and principally directed toward elimination and expurgation of an imaginary morbific substance, and that the indication most frequently to be followed was, to scatter and set in motion the morbific accumulation, and to provide for its expulsion through the salivary and tracheal glands, perspiration, and urine; to purify the blood by potions of roots and herbs (Wurzel und Holztränke), regarded as rational and obedient servants in removing morbific matters (acrids and impurities) *which never existed;* furthermore, to draw off mechanically this fictitious matter by setons, fontanels, and by keeping up constant local discharges from the skin with blisters and bark of spurge-laurel; but the chief indication was to throw off and purge away the *materia peccans* or noxious substances, as they were called, through the intestinal canal by means of laxatives and purgatives, often dignified by the appellation of *solvents* (of infarctions?) *and gentle aperients*, for the sake of seeming more profoundly significant, and giving them a more flattering appearance. Such were the measures employed in the removal of hostile pathogenetic substances, that never were, nor could have been present in the production or maintenance of diseases as they occur in the human organism, living by virtue of a spiritual principle; diseases that never could have been of other nature than that of a dynamic derangement of life in regard to its sensations and functions.[13]

Now, if we admit, what cannot be doubted, that no disease (unless occasioned by entirely indigestible, or other hurtful matter, swallowed or lodged in the primæ viæ, or other apertures and cavities of the body, or caused, *e. g.*, by a foreign substance penetrating the skin) can be derived from the presence of any material substance, but that each disease is always and only a special, virtual, and dynamical discordancy of our sensorial condition (health), how inappropriate, then, it must appear to any reasonable man to make use of a curative method, directed toward the evacuation[14] of those fictitious matters, since in the principal diseases of mankind, viz., the chronic, nothing is gained, but much harm always done by such measures!

In short, it cannot be denied that these degenerated matters and impurities, becoming visible in disease, are nothing but productions of the diseased organism itself, laboring under abnormal functional derangement, and that they are frequently expelled by the organism with violent—and even too violent—an action, without the aid of purgatives; notwithstanding which, new quantities of refuse matter are formed as long as the organism continues to suffer from this disease. These substances present themselves to the true physician as symptoms of the disease, and aid him in recognizing the nature and image of the same, in order to cure it by means of a similar medicinal morbific potency (Krankheits-Potenz). The modern representatives of the old school, however, no longer wish to appear as if their object in curing were the expulsion of morbific material. They declare their numerous and various evacuants to be employed in accordance with *a derivative* method of cure, as an example of which; they regard the natural spontaneous efforts of the diseased organism to re-establish health, by terminating fevers through perspiration and urine; stitches in the side by nosebleed, sweating, and expectoration of mucus; other diseases by vomiting, diarrhœa, or hæmorrhage from the anus; arthritic pains by sanious ulcers of the leg; inflammation of the throat by salivation, etc., or by means of metastases and abscesses, called forth by nature in parts remote from the seat of disease.

For these reasons they considered it their wisest course to *imitate* nature by approaching most diseases in a circuitous way, after the manner of the vital force when left to itself. For these reasons they employed indirect,[15] stronger, heterogeneous irritation in parts remote from the seat of disease, caused evacuations in organs least related (dissimilar) to the diseased structures, and maintained these in order, as it were, to *divert* the disease in that direction.

This derivation was, and continued to be, one of the chief curative methods of the prevailing school of medicine.

In this imitation of nature in the act of relieving herself, as others express it, they endeavored forcibly to excite new symptoms in structures least affected by the disease, and better able to bear drug effects, with the intention of diverting[16] the primary disease, apparently in the form of critical excretions, thus permitting the curative powers of nature[17] to perform the gradual resolution (*lysis*).

This was executed by resorting to diaphoretics and diuretics, venesections, setons, and fontanels; but most frequently by irritant evacuants applied to the œsophagus or intestinal canal, acting as emetics in their upward, and as cathartics in their downward action; being employed most frequently in the latter manner, they were also known as aperients and solvents.[18]

By way of assisting this derivative method, the counter-irritants related to the former were employed, such as sheep's wool worn next to the skin, footbaths, nauseants; furthermore, the stomach and intestines were tormented by hunger (hunger-cure), or by remedies producing pain, inflammation, and suppuration in proximate or remote parts, such as horse-radish and mustard-poultices, plaster of cantharides, spurge-laurel, setons (fontanels), Authenrieth's salve (tartar emetic ointment), moxa, the hot iron, acupuncture, etc.; all done in imitation of the crude efforts of nature, who, when left to her own resources, endeavors to free herself from dynamic disease by creating pain in remote parts by metastases and abscesses; by producing eruptions and running sores, all of no avail if the disease is chronic.

Obviously, therefore, no rational grounds, but rather the convenience of curing by imitation, governed the old school in using these absurd, pernicious, and indirect methods of cure, derivative, as well as counter-irritant, and induced its adoption of these unserviceable, debilitating, and injurious processes, by which disease was for a time apparently ameliorated or relieved, inasmûch as another more serious malady was called forth in its place. Can such destructive measures be properly termed a cure?

The old school merely followed the rude instinctive example of nature in her inadequate[19] endeavors at resistance, when directed against moderately acute affections. They only copied the sustaining power of life (Lebens-Erhaltungs-Kraft), which, incapable of exercising reason if left to itself in diseases, and resting entirely upon the organic laws of the body, acts alone according to these laws, without reason or deliberation. They followed crude nature, who cannot, like a skilful surgeon, heal a wound by first intention by coadapting its gaping edges; who does not know how to adjust and replace the divergent ends of a fractured bone, notwithstanding her ability to furnish (often superabundantly) osseous matter; who cannot tie a wounded artery, but exhausts all her energy in causing the wounded person to bleed to death; who does not know how to reduce a dislocated humerus, but, on the contrary, prevents human art from accomplishing reduction by speedily producing a swelling around the joint; who, in order to remove a splinter from the cornea, destroys the whole eye by suppuration; who, in spite of her display of energy, reduces a strangulated inguinal hernia by nothing less than mortification of the intestines and death; and who, by transposing morbid processes (Metaschematismen) in dynamic diseases, often increases the misery of the sick. Nay, this unreasonable vital force rashly receives into the body those chronic miasms (psora, syphilis, sycosis), the greatest tormentors of our earthly existence, the source of innumerable diseases, under which humanity groans for hundreds, nay, for thousands of years, and unable even to palliate one of these, this same vital force is utterly incapable of removing such diseases from the organism of its own accord, but suffers them to rankle in the system, until death closes the eyes of the sufferer after a long life of sorrow.

How could the old school, calling itself rational, be justified in choosing this unintelligent vital force, this blind guide, as its best instructor in an office of such high importance as that of healing, requiring so much thought and power of judgment? How dared it imitate, without hesitation, all those indirect and revolutionary processes inaugurated in diseases by that vital force, and copy them as if they were the *non plus ultra*, the best that reason could devise? Did not God grant us his noblest gift, reflecting reason and unfettered power of deliberation in order that we might, for the benefit of mankind, surpass immeasurably the effort of the unguided vital power in bringing relief?

If, therefore, the ordinary school of medicine, in its rash imitation of crude, unreasonable, automatic vital energy, attacks the unoffending parts and organs with its curative methods of counter-irritation and derivation (its usual course of procedure), torturing them with overpowering pain, or, more commonly, by forcing them to waste their strength and substance in evacuations, that school strives to divert the morbid vital activity from the originally affected portions to those artificially attacked, thus, by means of a circuitous, debilitating, and generally painful process, indirectly endeavoring to compel the natural disease to vanish, and trying to supplant it by a far greater heterogeneous disease in healthier parts.[20]

Indeed, the disease, if acute, and consequently destined to be of short duration, will vanish, even during these heterogeneous attacks upon remote and dissimilar parts, but it will not have been cured. There is nothing deserving the distinguished title of a *cure* in this revolutionary* treatment, possessing no direct immediate pathological bearing upon the structures primarily affected. It may be confidently assumed that the acute disease would have vanished of its own accord, and certainly sooner, without such serious assault upon sound vital parts, and without after-effects and less waste of strength. Neither the course adopted by crude natural force, nor the allopathic copy of the latter can bear comparison with the direct dynamic (homœopathic) treatment, which, without waste of strength, rapidly extinguishes the disease.

But in by far the greatest proportion of cases of disease, known as chronic, these impetuous, weakening, and indirect therapeutic measures of the old school scarcely ever prove to be of the least benefit. For a few days at most they suspend one or another of those troublesome manifestations of disease which return, however, as soon as nature has become inured to that counter-stimulus; and the disease will reappear with more violence, because the vital powers have been reduced by the pain[21] of counter-irritation and improper evacuations.

---

* Synonymous with revulsive, a more usual medical expression; Hahnemann probably intended to emphasize the idea by using the word "revolutionär."—TRANSLATOR.

While most physicians of the old school, *imitating in a general manner* the spontaneous curative efforts of crude nature abandoned to her own resources, arbitrarily exercised in their practice this nominally useful mode of derivation (whenever an illusory indication seemed to demand it), others aiming at a still higher object, and seeing the incipient struggles of nature for relief in spontaneous and antagonistic metastases, they undertook to accelerate and increase these efforts by means of evacuants and derivatives, supposing that by virtue of their pernicious measures they were acting under the guidance of nature (*duce natura*), and that they were entitled to the exalted name of servants of nature (*ministri naturæ*).

Having observed that in protracted diseases such evacuations, induced by the vitality of the patient, were frequently attended by brief remissions of severe pains, paralysis, convulsions, etc., the old school regarded these derivative actions as the true way to be followed, and therefore accelerated, maintained, and increased them in attempting to cure diseases. But they never discovered that all such evacuations and secretions (seemingly critical), called forth by the spontaneous efforts of nature in chronic diseases, only procured palliative and brief alleviation, adding so little to an actual cure, that their influence amounted rather to an aggravation of the original internal malady, by wasting strength and substance. No patient suffering from a protracted malady, was ever known to have regained permanent health by those rude efforts of nature, nor any chronic disease to have been cured by those evacuations, resulting from the action[22] of the organism. But on the contrary, after a brief respite, the original evil in such cases evidently increases; the duration of its remissions grow constantly shorter and shorter, while the painful periods of aggravation return with more frequency and violence, in spite of the continued evacuations.

The same result may be observed when nature, abandoned to her own resources, in struggling with the dangers of an internal chronic affection, has no other way of safety than that of producing external local symptoms, for the purpose of diverting the danger from parts indispensable to life, and directing them to structures of less vital importance (metastasis). Hence, those procedures of the energetic vital force being devoid of reason, reflection, or precaution, will never lead to actual relief or to a real cure; they are mere brief, palliative respites in the dangerous course of the inner disease, at the sacrifice of much strength and substance, without diminishing the primitive disease in the least degree. These measures, at most, are able to postpone dissolution which, without the intervention of a genuine homœopathic cure, would be the inevitable result.

From the allopathic point of view held by the old school, those rude, automatic efforts of nature were not only greatly overestimated, but totally misinterpreted as genuine curative agencies; they were increased and accelerated under the vain hope of destroying and radically curing the entire evil. Whenever, in cases of chronic disease, one or another of the intolerable symptoms of the inner disease appeared to be relieved by efforts of vitality, producing, for example, a moist eruption on the skin, in that case the servant of rude nature (*minister naturæ*) would place a plaster of cantharides, or an exutorium (spurge-laurel) upon the ichorous surface, in order to draw out more humor (moisture) from the skin (*duce natura*), for the purpose of assisting and supporting the purpose of nature (by removing the morbific matter from the body ?). But sometimes, if the effect of the remedy proved to be too intense, the moist eruption too inveterate, and the body too irritable, that servant of nature had only increased the external affection considerably, without benefit to the primitive disease. He aggravated the pains, which deprived the sufferer of sleep, and reduced his strength (or even brought on a febrile or malignant form of erysipelas). At other times, by gently acting upon the local disease (perhaps yet recent), by a kind of improper, superficial homœopathism, he would thus drive away from its site that local symptom, set up by nature on the skin for the relief of the inner more dangerous evil; but he thereby increased the latter, and induced the vital powers to institute a more serious metaschematism towards other and more vital parts. In place of those local symptoms, the patient then suffered from dangerous inflammation of the eyes, deafness, cramps of the stomach, epileptiform spasms, attacks of asthma, apoplexy, or mental disorders, etc.[23]

Acting under the same delusion of assisting the vital forces in their curative endeavors, that *minister naturæ* applied numerous leeches, in case the diseased force of nature caused congestion of the rectum or anus (blind piles), hoping to furnish an outlet for the blood in that place. The result would be a brief and scarcely noticeable improvement, but with loss of bodily strength, giving rise to more violent congestion to those parts, without lessening the original disease in the least degree.

In nearly every case where the morbid vitality strove to evacuate a little blood by means of emesis or cough, etc., in order to allay a dangerous internal affection, the old school physician hastened to assist (*duce natura*) those supposed curative efforts of nature by copious abstraction of blood from a vein; but never without evil consequences in the future, or without evident debilitation of the body.

In order to promote the intentions of nature, the old school physician was in the habit of treating cases of chronic nausea by causing profuse evacuations from the stomach, by administering powerful emetics—never with a beneficial, but often with evil result; not infrequently with dangerous and even fatal consequences.

To relieve an internal morbid condition, the vital force sometimes produces violent swellings of external glands, in which event that pretended servant of nature entertains the hope of assisting her purposes by inflaming those swellings by all sorts of stimulating ointments and plasters, and then opening the ripe abscess by incision, to allow the escape of the offending morbific matter (?). But experience furnishes hundreds of proofs of the protracted mischief resulting unexceptionally from such proceedings.

Having frequently observed in chronic disorders slight alleviation of great distress, following spontaneous night-sweats, or loose alvine discharges, the old school practitioner considers himself bound to follow and promote these hints of nature (*duce natura*) by instituting and maintaining copious perspirations, or by subjecting his patient for years to a course of so-called gentle laxatives, in order to sustain and increase those efforts of nature (the vital force of the unintelligent organism) leading, as he thinks, to the cure of the entire chronic disorder, and to the more speedy liberation of the patient from his disease (the substance causing the disease?).

But the result is always contrary to the intention: aggravation of the original complaint.

In accordance with his preconceived, though groundless opinions, the physician of the old school persists in his process of promoting[24] those endeavors of morbid vitality, and of increasing those ever ruinous and never salutary derivative and evacuant efforts of the patient's system. He does not perceive that all above-named local symptoms, evacuations, and apparent derivative actions (begun and supported by the unthinking, unguided vital force in conquering the original chronic disease) are in fact the disease itself, and the signs of the entire disorder, for the cure of which, a homœopathic medicine, selected in accordance with its similitude of effect, would have been the most successful and speedy remedy.

Since the crude efforts of nature for attaining relief in acute, and more particularly in chronic diseases, are extremely imperfect and in themselves a disease, it was readily to be understood that the artificial furtherance of these efforts would only increase the difficulty; to say the least, it would not be an improvement on the spontanecons efforts of nature in the case of acute affections. The vital power in producing its crises, moves in obscure ways which medical art was incompetent to follow; therefore the latter only undertakes to reach its object from without by violent remedies, much less beneficial, but on the contrary, far more aggravating and debilitating than the means employed by the instinctive, unguided vital force left to itself. Not even that imperfect kind of relief, induced by natural derivatives and crises, can be produced by allopathy in a similar manner; that school will find itself greatly outdone, even by curative measures as imperfect as those of vitality left to itself.

By the use of lacerating implements it was attempted to produce nosebleed in imitation of the natural kind, for the purpose of relieving, for example, attacks of chronic headache. Although blood was made to flow abundantly from the nasal cavities, depriving the patient of strength, yet the relief thus obtained amounted to nothing, or was, at least, far more insignificant than if, at other times, but a few drops were shed by the instinctive and spontaneous impulses of the vital force.

So-called critical perspiration or diarrhœa, caused by the ever active vital force after sudden attacks of sickness, occasioned by mental agitation, fright, strains, or cold, will remove these acute affections, though temporarily, with far more efficacy than all the sudorifics or cathartics obtained from the apothecary-shop, which increase the trouble, as daily experience teaches.

The vital force, capable of acting only in harmony with the physical arrangement of our organism, and without reason, insight, or reflection, was not given to us that we should regard it as the best guide in the cure of diseases (Krankheits-Heilerin), having the power of reducing those sad deviations from health to their normal standard; and still less was that vital force given to us, that its imperfect and morbid efforts (to rescue itself from disease) might be imitated by servile physicians, adopting methods more inappropriate and depressing than those of the vital force itself; nor that indolent physicians might be enabled to spare themselves all intellectual effort, reflection, and consideration, necessary for the discovery and practice of the noblest of human arts, the true art of healing, instead of contenting themselves with imperfect imitation of the crude curative efforts of unintelligent nature, and then proclaiming theirs as the "rational art of healing."

What man of sense would undertake to imitate nature in her endeavors of coming to the rescue? Those efforts are, in fact, the disease itself; and the morbidly affected vital force is the producer of disease becoming manifest. Necessarily, therefore, every artificial imitation as well as the suppression of these natural efforts must either increase the evil, or render it dangerous by suppression; the allopathist does both, and then extols this practice as healing art, as "rational" healing art!

He is in the wrong. *That noble innate power, destined to govern life in the most perfect manner during health*, equally present in all parts of the organism, in the sensitive as well as in the irritable fibre; that untiring mainspring of all normal, natural, bodily functions, was never created for the purpose of aiding itself in diseases, nor to exercise a healing art worthy of imitation. *No! The true healing art is that intellectual office incumbent on the higher human mind, and free powers of thought, discriminating and deciding according to causes; a duty of which office is, whenever that instinctive, unconscious, and unreasoning, but automatic, energetic vital force has been thrown into discordant action by disease, to harmonize those discordancies by means of a similar pathogenetic affection of higher degree, originated by a drug homœopathically selected; after this, the natural morbid affection will no longer be able to act upon the vital force, which will get rid of the former, while the latter merely continues to be engaged with the similar, rather more powerful pathogenetic drug affection, against which it may now direct its entire energy; ere long the drug affection will be overcome, leaving the vital power free and able to return to its normal condition of health, and to its destination: "to animate the organism and maintain its health," without having suffered painful or debilitating onslaughts during these transformations. How to reach this result is taught by the homœopathic healing art.*

Not a few patients, however, treated according to the abovenamed methods of the old school, escaped from their diseases, not the chronic (unvenereal) kinds, but merely from the acute, less dangerous forms; and this was accomplished by means so painful, circuitous, and often so imperfect that such treatment could not properly be called a cure accomplished by gentle means. By abstracting blood, or by suppressing one of the main symptoms through the agency of an enantiopathic, palliative remedy (*contraria contrariis*), those less dangerous cases of acute disease were kept under, or suspended by means of counter-stimulants and derivatives (antagonistic and revellent remedies) directed to parts remote from the seat of disease, up to the time at which the brief illness would have terminated its natural course. These circuitous proceedings deprived the patient of strength and substance to such a degree, that the greater and better part of the work of completing the cure of the disease, of restoring the wasted strength and substance of the patient, was left to nature's supporting power of life; this, besides conquering the natural acute disease, had now the superadded burden of overcoming the consequences of improper treatment. In less dangerous cases the power of nature succeeded by its own energy, however laboriously, imperfectly, and under great difficulties, gradually to restore the functions to their normal condition.

It remains highly dubious whether the natural process of recovery is really shortened or assisted in the least by the interference of the old practice in cases of acute disease; since neither physician nor nature could act otherwise than indirectly, excepting that the derivative and antagonistic appliances of the former are much more severe and weakening than the processes of the latter.

The old school possesses still another curative process,[25] called the *stimulating* and *tonic* method (by means of *excitants, nervines, tonics, comfortants, roborants*). It is surprising that they should boast of this mode of treatment.

Has the old school, notwithstanding its frequent attempts, ever been able to remedy the bodily weakness, caused, kept up, and increased by a chronic disease, by prescribing ethereal Rhenish wine or fiery Tokay? In such cases strength would only be more and more reduced (since the origin of debility, the chronic disease, had not been cured), in proportion to the quantity of wine which the patient had been ordered to consume; because, in the secondary action of the vital force, debility succeeds artificial excitement.

Or was strength ever restored by Cinchona bark in any of these numerous cases, or by those ill-understood, ambiguous substances known as *bitters*, so hurtful in many other respects? Have not these vegetable substances, together with the preparations of iron, declared under all circumstances to be tonic and strengthening, added new diseases to the older ones, by virtue of their peculiar pathogenetic properties, without mitigating the debility, dependent on inveterate and unknown disease of long standing?

Was an incipient paralysis of an arm or a leg (commonly produced by a chronic malady) ever diminished in the least, or with any degree of permanency by those so-called *unguenta nervina*, or any of the other ethereal or balsamic inventions, without the previous eradication of the malady itself? Or have electric and voltaic shocks ever produced any other effects[26] upon such limbs beyond increasing, or even completing, the paralysis and extinction of muscular activity, or the sensitiveness of nerves?

Have not those highly praised excitants and aphrodisiacs, such as amber, the smelt, tincture of cantharides, truffles, cardamom seeds, cinnamon, and vanilla, invariably produced complete impotence (always based upon a chronic miasm), when the sexual power had been previously weakened?

Why should an excitement or increase of strength, lasting a few hours, be looked upon as a success, when the subsequent result proves to be the permanent counterpart; when the evil has been rendered incurable, in accordance with the laws governing the action of all palliatives?

The slight benefit derived from excitants and roborants, during convalescence from acute diseases (treated in the old manner), was overbalanced a thousand times by the ill effects produced by these remedies in chronic diseases.

Whenever old medicine is at loss what to do in a tedious disease, it blindly blunders away with its so-called *alterative* remedies (*alterantia*); in that case the dreadful mercurials (calomel, corrosive sublimate, and mercurial ointment) are used as its chief remedies, which (in non-venereal diseases) are perniciously permitted to act upon the body in quantities, and for a length of time sufficient to undermine the health entirely. Great changes are truly wrought in this manner, but always of an evil kind, and health is always completely ruined by this extremely hurtful metal when its use is out of place.

Cinchona bark, specific as a homœopathic fever remedy only in genuine swamp-ague (provided it is used in the absence of psora), is now prescribed in massive doses in all epidemic intermittent fevers, often spread over large countries; herein the old school evinces its palpable rashness, for these fevers assume a different character every year, and therefore almost always demand for their removal another homœopathic remedy, which, if administered in one, or some few very minute doses, cures them radically in a few days. Since these epidemic fevers have regular periods of occurrence (type), and since only the type of these intermittent fevers is recognized by the old school, knowing no other fever remedy than Peruvian bark, nor desirous of knowing any other, that school, I say, in its monotonous routine, imagines that it has cured these fevers as long as the type of these epidemics can be suppressed by large doses of bark, or its expensive extract (quinia); (the irrational vital force proving wiser in this instance, often seeking to prevent this suppression for months). But the duped patient grows constantly worse after such a suppression of the periodicity (type) of his fever than he was during the attack itself. With sallow countenance, difficulty of breathing, constriction in the hypochondriac regions, disturbed digestion, and loss of appetite, without refreshing sleep, weak and listless, often with tense swelling of the legs, abdomen, or even of the face and hands, that patient creeps out of the hospital, *dismissed as cured,* and not infrequently years of laborious homœopathic treatment are required, perhaps not to heal and restore the health, but merely to continue the life of one of those patients, radically ruined (cured?), and made the victim of an artificial cachexia.

The old school delights in its ability to convert the stupor peculiar to typhoid fevers into a kind of temporary exhilaration by means of *valerian,* possessing antipathic properties in such cases; but since this exhilaration does not last, and another brief space of animation can only be gained by increased doses of valerian, the point is soon reached at which even the largest doses cease to act.

This palliative, after having excited the patient by its primary action, paralyzes the entire vital force by its secondary effect, thus insuring the speedy dissolution of the sufferer by means of this *rational mode of treatment* peculiar to the old school; none will escape from it. And still the followers of this routine-practice never learn to see how surely its treatment will prove fatal; because the fatal result is invariably ascribed to the malignancy of the disease.

A palliative that deserves to be dreaded by patients even more than the last is *Digitalis purpurea;* this was hitherto the pride of the old school when the too rapid and excited pulse, in chronic diseases, was to be compelled (in true symptomatic fashion) to beat more slowly. Although it is truly astonishing how this powerful remedy, by its enantiopathic effect, quiets the rapid, excited pulse, and how it diminishes the pulsation of the arteries in a marked degree, *for a few hours after the first dose;* yet soon the pulse will become rapid again. Now the dose is increased, that it may once more reduce its velocity a little, and it is reduced accordingly, but only for a shorter period than before, and so on, until the last and highest palliative doses cease to have any effect, and the pulse, no longer able to resist the after-effects of the foxglove, now becomes far more frequent than it was previous to the use of that herb; its beats can be counted no longer; sleep, appetite, and strength vanish, and—the patient pays the cost with his life; none will escape; death, or hopeless insanity[27] is the inevitable result.

This was the treatment of the allopathic physician. But the patients *were obliged* to conform to this deplorable necessity, because they fared no better at the hands of others of the same school, who had derived their knowledge from the same deceptive books.

The fundamental cause of chronic diseases (non-venereal), together with their remedies, remained unknown to those practitioners, vainly boasting of causal cures, and their diagnosis founded on the investigation into the genesis of the disease. How dared they attempt the eradication of that long list of chronic diseases with their indirect measures, their pernicious imitations of the irrational vital force in its spontaneous struggles for relief, never intended as a model for the treatment of diseases?

Mistaking the imaginary character of the disease for the cause, they directed their radical curative measures against cramp, inflammation (plethora), fever, general and partial debility, mucus, putrefaction, infarctions, etc., all of which they thought themselves able to remove by means of their (superficially known) antagonistic remedies, such as antispasmodics, antiphlogistics, tonics, stimulants, antiseptics, solvents, percutients, derivatives, and evacuants.[28]

Curative drugs, however, can never be found if searched for under the guidance of such general indications, especially in the common Materia Medica of the old school, based, as I have shown elsewhere,[29] mostly upon conjectures and false conclusions, *ab usu in morbis*, and mingled with falsehood and deceit.

With an equal degree of recklessness they waged war against still more hypothetical so-called indications, such as deficiency or surplus of oxygen, nitrogen, carbon or hydrogen in the juices; or against increased or diminished susceptibility of the sensitive sphere, or of reproduction; against arterial, venous, and capillary engorgement, asthenia, etc., without due knowledge of the means of cure applicable to so fanciful an object. This was mere ostentation; treatment to be sure, but not for the benefit of the patient.

The last vestige of the apparent propriety of that kind of treatment was destroyed by the *ancient custom, now even made obligatory, of compounding drugs in form of a recipe.* The true action of these medicinal substances, ever and unexceptionally varying from each other in effect, was almost entirely unknown. In preparing a recipe, some drug (unknown as to the scope of its pathogenetic effects) is placed at the head of the list, as principal remedy (*basis*), in order to conquer what the physician considers as the principal character of the disease; then one or more remedies (equally unknown as to the scope of their effects) are added either for the purpose of removing certain accessory indications, or by way of assistance to the rest (*adjuvantia*); finally, a third substance (the limits of whose action are equally unknown) is introduced, in order to correct the effect of the others (*corrigens*); whereupon the whole is mixed (decocted, extracted); or, perhaps, put in shape, combined with a medicated syrup of different quality, or distilled medicated water; all this is done under the impression, that each of these component parts (ingredients) would fulfil in the body of the patient the duty assigned to it in the imagination of the prescriber, without being disturbed or confused by the other things in the mixture, as should reasonably be expected. One of these ingredients must partially or wholly cancel the effect of the other, or impart to it or to the remainder a different, unexpected mode of action and direction, thus making it *impossible* to obtain the desired effect. The result was frequently of a kind which neither was nor could have been anticipated from one of these inexplicably enigmatic mixtures; it appeared in the form of a *new modification of disease*, frequently obscured by the tumult of morbid symptoms, but finally assuming a permanent form under the prolonged use of the recipe. The result, then, is an additional artificial disease, complicated with the original one, an aggravation of the original malady. Or, supposing the recipe had not been frequently repeated, but to have been exchanged for one or more new prescriptions of other ingredients, in quick succession, a greater sinking of strength would, at least, have ensued; because the prescribed remedies neither had, nor were intended to have, any direct pathological relation to the original disease; they only uselessly and perniciously attacked the parts least affected by the disease.

To witness the unreasonable process of mixing in one formula several drugs, even if the effect of each upon the human body had been well known (the writer of a recipe frequently does not know even the thousandth part of this effect), to mix a variety of such ingredients, several of which are themselves of a manifold, composite kind, and whose individual and special effect is scarcely known, but always different from that of the rest, and then, to see such an incomprehensible mixture administered to the patient in large and frequent doses, all in the vain hope of establishing a certain designed curative effect—such, I say, must arouse indignation in the mind of every thinking and unbiassed[30] observer.

The result is, of course, contrary to any definite expectation. Although changes and effects do occur, they are badly adapted to the purpose, hurtful, and pernicious.

Who would apply the name of *cure* to this blundering interference with a diseased human body?

A cure may be expected only through the aid of the remnant

of vitality led into the right path of activity by an appropriate remedy, but never by an artificial, debilitating process, pushed to the verge of endurance. And yet, the old school knows no other way to manage inveterate disorders, than to belabor the patient with all sorts of tormenting, debilitating, and even fatal remedies. Can that school save while it destroys? Does this practice deserve any other name than that of a pernicious art (Unheilkunst)? It acts, *lege artis*, as contrary to this purpose as possible, and performs (it almost seems as if *by design*) ἀλλοῖα, that is, the opposite of what it should perform. Does this merit our praise? Shall we endure this longer?

In modern times old physic finally has overstepped all bounds in its cruelty and impropriety of action towards suffering fellow-men, as every impartial observer must admit, and as physicians of that school itself (such as Krüger-Hansen), prompted by conscience, were obliged to acknowledge to the world.

It was high time that the allwise Creator and Benefactor of mankind commanded these horrors to cease, set a limit to these tortures, and called into existence a healing art which, as the opposite of the former, should save the strength of the patient as much as possible, and restore his health directly, quickly, and permanently, by means of mild and few remedies which should have been previously well considered and thoroughly proved according to their effect, and administered in the finest doses, according to the only natural law of cure: *similia similibus curantur;* without wasting the vital force and substance by emetics, protracted sweeping out of the bowels, warm baths, sudorifics or salivation; without shedding the heart's blood, and without weakening and torturing by painful revulsives; without burdening the sufferer to the verge of incurability with new chronic drug diseases, by assiduously urging the use of wrong debilitating medicines of qualities unknown to the prescriber; without the abuse of violent palliatives, according to the motto: *contraria contrariis,* thus placing the horse behind the cart, after the fashion of merciless routine that leads the way to the grave instead of recovery. It was high time that God mercifully permitted homœopathy to be discovered.

Through observation, thought, and experience, I learned that contrary to old allopathy, the best way to cure is to be found by following the proposition: *In order to cure gently, quickly, unfailingly, and permanently, select for every case of disease a medicine, capable of calling forth by itself an affection similar* (ὅμοιον πάθος) *to that which it is intended to cure!*

Hitherto none *taught* this homœopathic method of cure, no one put it in practice. But if the truth is contained alone in this process, as others will observe like myself, then we must expect to discover[31] its actual traces in all past ages, although it was not acknowledged for thousands of years.

And such is actually the case. In all ages those sufferers *who were really cured* rapidly, permanently, and visibly *through medicines,* were cured alone (though without the knowledge of the physician) by a (homœopathic) remedy, possessing the power of producing by itself a similar morbid condition, provided these patients did not, perchance, recover through the agency of some other beneficial circumstance, or through spontaneous termination of the disease, or in the length of time by virtue of their physical power of endurance, tried under allopathic, antagonistic treatment; for a direct cure differs widely from recovery gained by an indirect course.

Even those actual cures produced, however rarely, by a variety of compounded drugs, will be found to result from the predominant remedy which was of homœopathic nature.

A still more striking proof may be seen in those instances where physicians had, contrary to custom (hitherto admitting only medicinal mixtures in the form of recipes), now and then effected a speedy cure by means of a simple drug. There we may see with astonishment that the result was always due to a medicine capable of producing *by itself* an affection similar to the disease in which it was used, although the physicians themselves did not know what they did, laboring under a spell of forgetfulness of the opposite doctrines of their school. They prescribed a remedy, the exact opposite of which they should have used according to the rules of their customary therapeutics; but *in this manner only* were the patients cured quickly.[32]

Without counting those cases where popular empiricism (not their own inventiveness) had furnished physicians with specific remedies for diseases of unvarying character, enabling them to cure in a direct manner—for instance, venereal chancre-disease with quicksilver; disease resulting from contusions, by arnica; intermittent fevers of marshy districts, by Peruvian bark; recent cases of itch, by flowers of sulphur, etc.—without counting these instances, we find that all other modes of treatment used by old-school physicians in chronic diseases, are, without exception, merely pernicious and debilitating tortures, aggravating the sufferings of the patient. Such are the measures practiced with an air of superiority, and at a ruinous expense to the patient.

Sometimes accidental experience would lead them to homœopathic treatment,[33] but still they did not recognize the law of nature, according to which such cures were and must be brought about.

It is, therefore, of extreme importance for the welfare of mankind, to seek out the causes of these rare and highly salutary cures. The disclosures made with regard to them are of the highest significance. Such cures never were effected by other means than by homœopathic remedies, possessing the power of producing a disease similar to that which was to be cured. Such curative results were speedily and permanently produced by medicines that fell, as by accident, into the hands of medical prescribers, who used them in violation of customary systems and therapeutics (often without really knowing what they did, and why), but who unintentionally established the actual existence of a natural law of cure, that is of homœopathy, which had hitherto been left undiscovered in the past ages of medicine, blinded by prejudices, notwithstanding numerous facts and indications pointing in that direction.

Even in the domestic practice of non-professional classes of people, gifted with sound sense and the faculty of observation, this mode of healing has been found by manifold experience to be the most safe, thorough, and reliable.

Recently frozen limbs are covered with frozen sauerkraut or rubbed with snow.[34]

An experienced cook holds his scalded hand at a small distance from the fire, without heeding the primary aggravation of the pain, taught by experience that in a short time, often in a few minutes, he can restore the appearance of healthy, painless skin to the burnt spot.[35]

Other sensible laymen, such as japanners, treat a burn with a remedy capable of exciting a similar *burning* sensation, *e. g.*, strong and well-warmed alcohol,[36] or oil of turpentine,[37] thereby restoring the parts to health in the course of a few hours; well aware that cooling salves would not accomplish the same object in as many months, and that cold water[38] would increase the evil.

The old and experienced reaper, without being addicted to the use of brandy, will never drink cold water (*contraria contrariis*) whenever he has become heated in the sun to a degree approaching high fever. Knowing the danger likely to follow such an attempt, he takes a small quantity of some heating fluid, a mouthful of brandy, for instance; experience, the teacher of truth, having convinced him of the advantage and efficacy of this homœopathic measure by which heat, as well as fatigue, is speedily removed.[39]

Indeed there have been physicians from time to time, who had *presentiments* that medicines, by their power of producing analogous morbid symptoms, would cure analogous morbid conditions.[40]

The author of one of the books ascribed to Hippocrates, *περὶ τόπων τῶν κατ' ἄνθρωπον*,[41] has these remarkable words: *διὰ τὰ ὅμοια νοῦσος γίνεται καὶ διὰ τὰ ὅμοια προσφερόμενα ἐκ νοσεύντων ὑγιαίνονται, διὰ τὸ ἐμέειν ἔμετος παύεται.*[42]

The truth of homœopathy has also been felt and expressed by physicians of later times. Thus, *e. g.*, Boulduc recognizes the fact that the purging quality of rhubarb is the cause of its power to allay diarrhœa.

Detharding conjectures[43] that colic in adults is mitigated by the infusion of senna, by virtue of its analogous effect of producing colic in the healthy.

Bertholon[44] confesses that electricity deadens and annuls, in disease, pain very similar in kind to that produced by electricity.

Thiury testifies that positive electricity, though in itself it accelerates the pulse, nevertheless retards it when accelerated by disease.[45]

Von Stœrck[46] expresses the idea: "If the thorn-apple deranges the mind, and produces insanity in the healthy, might it not, by changing the current of ideas, restore soundness of mind to the insane?"

Stahl, a Danish military physician, has expressed his conviction on this subject most distinctly. He says: "The rule accepted in medicine to cure by contraries is entirely wrong (*contraria contrariis*); he is convinced, on the contrary, that diseases vanish and are cured by means of medicines capable of producing a similar affection (*similia similibus*)." Thus burns are cured by approaching the fire; frozen limbs by the application of snow or very cold water; inflammation and contusions, by distilled spirits. In this manner he is in the habit of curing habitual acidity of the stomach most successfully by means of a very small dose of sulphuric acid, in cases where quantities of absorbing powders have been used in vain.

So near had the great truth sometimes been approached! But only a hasty thought was here and there bestowed upon it, and hence the indispensable reformation of the ancient way of treating disease, the conversion of the traditional defective manner of treatment, into a genuine, true, and certain art of healing, remain unaccomplished to the present day.

REMARKS

AND

EXPLANATORY NOTES TO THE REVIEW OF "PHYSIC," ETC.

---

[1] It would have been much more in accordance with sound common sense and the nature of the inquiry, if, for the purpose of treating a disease, they had sought for its primary cause as the *causa morbi*. In that case the method of cure which had proved efficacious in diseases produced by the same cause could have been successfully applied in all those of like origin, as, for instance, the same mercurial which is effectual in all venereal chancres is effectual also in any ulcer occurring on the glans penis after an impure connection. Had they discovered the primary cause of all other chronic (non-venereal) diseases to be a remote or recent infection by the itch-miasm (psora), and found for all these a common method of cure, one having due regard for the therapeutics of every individual case, according to which each and all of these chronic diseases could have been treated, then might they have boasted justly of having rightly apprehended and assumed as the basis of cure of chronic diseases, the only true and fruitful *causa morborum chronicorum* (non-venerorum), and that they could treat these diseases with the best success. But, ignorant of their origin from itch-miasm (first discovered by homœopathy, and subsequently provided with an effectual method of cure) they have, for many centuries, failed in curing all the countless chronic diseases. And yet they have boasted of aiming at the *prima causa*, and of following the only rational method in their treatment, although they had not the remotest idea of the only available knowledge, that of the psoric origin of chronic diseases, all of which they bunglingly aggravated.

[2] Every physician who treats according to such generalities, however boldly he may assume the name of a homœopathist, remains neither more nor less than a generalizing allopathist, since homœopathy is absolutely inconceivable without the most precise individualization.

[3] Now called homœopathic.

[4] "Wherever experience had taught us the curative power of

homœopathic medicines, whose mode of action could not be explained, they were straightway declared to be specifics : an utterly meaningless term, by which all further inquiry was lulled to sleep. But the homogeneous or specific (homœopathic) stimulants have long been proscribed as most pernicious agents." Rau, *On the Homœopathic Method of Cure*. Heidelberg, 1824, pp. 101–2.

[5] Dr. Rau (*Ueber d. Werth d. homœop. Heilverfahrens*. Heidelberg, 1824, p. 176, et seq.), though not fully initiated into homœopathy at that time, was so thoroughly convinced of the dynamic origin of even these fevers, that he treated them by one or two minute doses of homœopathic medicine without the least resort to evacuants. He relates two remarkable cases.

[6] In case of a sudden derangement of the stomach, marked by constant and offensive eructations tasting of tainted food, and usually accompanied by depression of spirits, cold hands and feet, the efforts of the ordinary practitioner have been directed altogether against the vitiated contents of the stomach, using active emetics to effect their complete expulsion. This end has been usually gained by tartar emetic with or without ipecac. But will the patient be found well and cheerful immediately afterwards ? By no means. Commonly such gastric disturbances are of *dynamic origin*, and are called forth by disturbing emotions (grief, fright, vexation) immediately after even a moderate meal. These two drugs are neither suited to the purpose of subduing this dynamic derangement, nor the revulsive emesis to which it gives rise. But, by producing their peculiar morbific symptoms, they will have aggravated the patient's condition, and the secretion of bile will have been deranged, so that he will find himself suffering for several days from the effects of this pretended causal cure, notwithstanding the violent and complete emptying of the contents of the stomach. But, if in place of using such powerful and injurious evacuants, the patient will apply but once, by olfaction, the highly diluted juice of pulsatilla (smelling of a globule no larger than a mustard-seed, moistened with the same), it will relieve the derangement of his condition in general, and that of his stomach in particular, and restore him in two hours. Should eructations still occur subsequently they will be only of tasteless and odorless gas ; the contents of the stomach will no longer be vitiated, his usual appetite will make its appearance with the return of the next meal, and he is well and cheerful. This is a real causal cure ; the other imaginary one is only a pernicious strain upon the patient's constitution.

The stomach, even if surcharged with indigestible food, scarcely ever requires a medicinal emetic. Nature possesses the best means of throwing off any superfluities by means of nausea, loathing, and even vomiting, perhaps with the assistance of mechanical measures, such as tickling the palate and fauces, thereby avoiding all the incidental effects of medicinal emetics; any remaining particles in the stomach will be assisted in passing downwards by a little decoction of coffee.

Supposing, however, that after overloading the stomach, its power of reaction were insufficient to produce vomiting, while, at the same time, the inclination to vomit had become extinct in consequence of excessive pain in the epigastrium, such an emetic would be followed by a dangerous or even fatal inflammation of the bowels, if administered during this paralyzed condition of the stomach. While a small quantity of strong coffee, frequently repeated, would have been sufficient to elevate dynamically the depressed susceptibility of the stomach, and to have enabled it to discharge without other aid, its superabundant contents by the mouth or rectum. Here the so-called causal cure is out of place.

In chronic diseases when accompanied by regurgitation of acrid gastric juice, the latter is forcibly and painfully removed by emetics, only to be replaced the next or the following days by gastric juice quite as acrid and even more abundant than the former. This would subside of its own accord, provided its dynamic cause were curatively annulled by a small dose of highly diluted sulphuric acid, or, if the acidity were of frequent occurrence, by the use of some other antipsoric remedy, corresponding to the rest of the symptoms. Of such pretended causal cures there are many in the old school, whose favorite occupation it is to clear out the material product of dynamic derangements by means of cumbersome and deleterious measures, without recognizing the dynamic source of the disorder, and without *curing* it rationally and homœopathically together with its products.

[7] Conditions which are dependent entirely upon psora, and easily cured by (dynamic) mild antipsoric remedies, without purging or vomiting.

[8] Notwithstanding that all hæmorrhages depend upon a dynamic alteration of vital force of health, the old school takes superabundance of blood to be their cause, and cannot refrain from venesections for the sake of getting rid of this supposed redundancy of vital juices. Afterwards the very evident and evil results, the depression of strength as well as the tendency or the actual transition into a typhoid state, is saddled upon the virulence of the disease, *which that school too often finds itself unable to cope with.* In fact, it persuades itself that it had performed a cure, according to the motto "*causam tolle,*" even if the patient does not recover, and in its way of speaking, all that was possible had been done for the patient whatever the result might be.

[9] Regardless of the probability that the human body has never contained one drop of blood too much, the old school regards a so-called plethoric condition as the material and chief cause of all hæmorrhages and inflammations, to be counteracted and removed by venesections and leeches. That is called rational treatment and causal cure. In general inflammatory fevers, and in acute pleurisy, physicians of the old school go so far as to call the coagulable lymph of the blood, the so-called buffy coat, the *materia peccans*, which they try to expel by repeated bloodlettings, notwithstanding its frequent reappearance with increased tenacity and firmness under renewed abstraction of blood. Thus blood is often shed until death is close at hand, if the inflammatory fever will not subside, in order to remove this buffy coat or supposed plethora. It never occurs to them that the inflamed blood is only the product of acute fever, *i. e.*, of the morbid, immaterial (dynamic) irritation, and that the latter is the sole cause of this great tumult in the arterial system, so easily subdued by the smallest dose of a homogeneous (homœopathic) remedy, for instance, by one small globule moistened with the decillionth dilution of aconite, at the same time avoiding vegetable acids, so that the *most violent pleuritic fever*, with all its threatening complications, is converted into health, *and cured in twenty-four hours* at most, *without bloodletting or any cooling medicines.* (A specimen of the patient's blood, taken from a vein, will no longer show a trace of buffiness.) While a patient afflicted with the same disease treated according to the "rational methods" of the old school, if, indeed, he escapes death for the present, after repeated bloodletting and unspeakable misery, will have to linger for many a sickly month, before his emaciated frame gains strength enough to stand erect, having narrowly escaped death from typhoid fever, leucophlegmasia, or suppurative disease of the lungs, the frequent consequence of such maltreatment.

He who has ever felt the pulse of a man an hour before the onset of the chills which always precede an attack of acute pleurisy, will be surprised when, two hours later, after the onset of the hot stage, he is to be persuaded of the necessity of resisting the present enormous plethora by frequent bloodletting, and he wonders by what miracle so many pounds of blood, now to be poured out, may have entered the patient's bloodvessels, felt quietly pulsating only two hours ago. Not one drachm more of blood can now roll through those vessels than they contained in times of health, or two hours earlier.

An allopathist, therefore, does not rid the fever-patient of a noxious superabundance of blood (which can never have existed), but robs him of his normal quantity of blood, necessary to life and recovery, and hence of strength—an enormous loss never to be repaired by medical aid. In the face of all this, these practitioners persist in the delusion of having acted in harmony with this (ill-conceived) motto, *causam tolle*, while in this case the cause of disease could never have consisted in a superabundance of blood, a thing without existence; here, on the contrary, the only true cause of disease was a morbid, dynamic inflammatory irritation of the vascular system, as has been and *will be proved in every case of the kind*, by the rapid and permanent cure effected as above related, by one or two incredibly fine and minute doses of aconite, possessing the power of homœopathically allaying such an irritation.

In a similar manner the old school misses its mark in its treatment of local inflammations by local depletion, particularly by the application of countless leeches, after the rash manner now inaugurated by Broussais. The palliative relief, primarily observed, is by no means crowned by a rapid and complete cure, because the ever remaining weakness and frailty of the part (often also the entire body) so treated, bears sufficient evidence that local inflammation was erroneously attributed to local plethora, and that the results of such local depletion are deplorable; for this virtually dynamic but apparently local inflammatory agency can be cancelled and cured by an equally fine dose of *aconite*, or the entire disorder may, if circumstances point that way, be permanently relieved by *belladonna*, without this wanton shedding of blood.

[10] Life was endangered when some pure water was injected into a vein (see Mullen, in Birch, *History of Royal Society*, vol. iv).

Atmospheric air injected into the bloodvessels proved fatal (see J. H. Voigt, *Magazine für den neuesten Zustand der Naturkunde*, I, III, p. 25).

[11] A girl, eight years of age, in Glasgow, bitten by a rabid dog, *had the wound immediately and thoroughly excised by the surgeon*, but nevertheless had hydrophobia thirty-six days afterwards, and died in two days. (*Med. Comment. on Edinb.*, Dec. ii, vol. ii, 1793.)

[12] In order to explain the origin of the large quantity of putrid matter and offensive ichor of sores, often observed in diseases, and in order to declare these appearances to be the exciting and maintaining matters of disease (notwithstanding the invisibility of miasms, or the impossible penetration of material substance into the body during infection), it was hypothetically asserted that the contagious matter, even if extremely fine, acted in the body like a ferment; that it vitiated the juices, changing them into a morbid ferment of its own kind, and maintaining the disease by virtue of its rank growth during the morbid process. What potent and ingeniously concocted purifying draughts could effect the elimination and separation from the human body of this inconstant process of reproduction, this mass of

so-called morbific matter, without leaving a vestige behind that might not, according to that hypothesis, again and again deteriorate and transform the juices into new morbific matters? In that case it were impossible to cure these diseases according to your method. It becomes evident that every hypothesis, no matter how skilfully worded, will lead to the most palpable inconsistencies, when it is not founded on truth. Syphilis of the most inveterate kind, if liberated from its frequent complication with psora, will be cured by means of one or two very minute doses of the decillionth dilution and potency of dissolved metallic quicksilver, after which the general syphilitic deterioration of the juices will be found to have been forever (dynamically) annihilated and dispelled.

[13] In that case every cold in the head, even the most protracted, must be invariably and speedily cured by careful blowing and cleansing of the nose.

[14] The expulsion of worms in so-called worm diseases has an appearance of necessity. But this appearance also is deceptive. Some lumbrical worms are perhaps to be found in many children, while the threadworm may be said to infest many others. But all of these, as well as a superabundance of one kind or another, invariably result from a general state of unhealthiness (psoric), combined with an improper mode of living. By improving the latter, and curing the psoric disease homœopathically, which is most easily accomplished during the period of childhood, no more worms will remain, and children cured in this manner will no longer be tormented by them, while they are rapidly reproduced in great numbers after the use of mere purgatives, even if these are compounded with wormseed (semen cinæ).

"But what of the tapeworm?" I hear them say; "must not this monstrous plague of mankind be expelled with all available force?"

Indeed, it is *sometimes* driven out, but not without much subsequent pain and danger to life. I would not burden my conscience with the death of so many hundreds of fellow-men, whose lives have been sacrificed by the use of the most debilitating, dreadful purgatives intended for the tapeworm; neither would I be guilty of the protracted illness of those who escaped death by purgation. Though continued for years, how seldom this purgative treatment, so destructive to health and life, attains its object, or if it succeed, does not the tapeworm as frequently reproduce itself?

What, if this forcible and often cruel and fatal method of expelling or killing these parasites were unnecessary?

The various species of tapeworm are only found in cases of psoric disease, and always disappear when that is cured. But before such cure can be accomplished, and during a period of comparative health, they do not inhabit the intestines proper, but rather the remnants of food and fecal matter contained therein, living quietly as in a world of their own, without causing the least inconvenience, finding their sustenance in the contents of the bowels. During this state they do not come in contact with the intestinal walls and remain harmless. But when from any cause a person is attacked by an acute disease, the contents of the bowels become offensive to the parasite, which, in its writhing and distress, touches and irritates the sensitive intestinal lining, thus increasing the complaints of the patient considerably by a particular kind of cramplike colic. (In a similar manner the fœtus in the womb becomes restless, twists its body, and moves whenever the mother is sick, but floats quietly in the liquor amnii, without distressing the mother, while she is well.)

It should be remarked, that the symptoms of a patient suffering from the above symptoms, are mostly of a kind that may be speedily (homœopathically) quieted by the most minute dose of the tincture of the root of the male fern, since the morbid condition of the patient, causing the disquietude of the parasite, is temporarily arrested by the remedy; the tapeworm is then quieted, and continues to live in the intestinal contents, without seriously disturbing the patient or his intestines, until the antipsoric cure has reached a stage, at which the psora has been so far extinguished that the fecal contents of the bowels cease to meet the wants of the worm, which now spontaneously departs from the convalescent patient forever, and without the least resort to purgatives.

[15] Instead of directly extinguishing the evil, quickly and without loss of strength and digression, by aiming homogeneous dynamic medicinal potencies at the diseased points of the organism, according to the usage of homœopathy.

[16] As if anything non-material could be eliminated by derivatives, directed against a material morbific substance, however subtile it is thought to be.

[17] Only moderately acute diseases are in the habit, so to say, of becoming neutralized (indifferenziren), and to terminate quietly with and without the application of the milder allopathic remedies. The vital power having rallied its strength, once more begins its normal sway where health has been disturbed by the storm of disease. But in the highly acute and in by far the most numerous affections of man, the chronic diseases, untutored nature, and the old school will be unsuccessful. There neither the vital force with its healing power, nor allopathy will effect a resolution; a truce perhaps may be the result,

giving the enemy time to rally his forces, and sooner or later to renew the assault with increased vigor.

[18] An expression betraying the presupposition and intention of expelling and dissolving some morbific substance.

[19] In ordinary practice it was customary to regard the cure of diseases by the spontaneous efforts of the nature of the organism, where no medicine was used, as model cures, worthy of imitation. *But it was a great error.* The lamentable and very imperfect attempts of vitality at self-redress in acute diseases, presents a spectacle calling for the exercise of compassion as well as of all the powers of our intelligent mind, in order to put an end to this self-torture by an actual, real cure. When a disease already present in the organism cannot be cured homœopathically by the power of nature applying another new, *similar* disease (§ 43–46), an opportunity rarely afforded (§ 50), and when the organism is left to its resources to conquer disease by its own strength and without external aid, its resistance being impotent in chronic miasms, we observe that these painful and often dangerous efforts of nature, instituted for the sake of relief at *any price*, frequently terminate by death this earthly existence.

As little as we mortals understand the economy of healthy life, and as surely as it must ever remain hidden from us, though plain to the all-seeing eye of the Creator and sustainer of his creatures, so impossible it will ever be for us to understand the internal processes of disturbed life in diseases. The internal process of diseases is only manifested by those observable changes, complaints, and symptoms, through which alone life expresses its inner disturbances; so that in every given case we must remain unable to determine which of the morbid symptoms are primary effects of the morbific agency (Schädlichkeit), or which are to be considered as the reaction of vital force in its spontaneous curative efforts. Both are seen to coalesce, and merely represent an outwardly reflected image of the totality of the inward disease, since the fruitless efforts of life, left to its own resources in terminating the disease, are themselves the disease of the entire organism. Consequently, more suffering than beneficent relief, often follows those evacuations called *crises*, commonly occurring toward the end of acute diseases. Whatever the vital force produces in these crises, and how it is produced will remain obscure, like all other inner processes of the organic economy of life. It is certain, however, that in all its exertions, the vital force *sacrifices and destroys a greater or less proportion of the affected parts*, in order to save the rest. This power of self-limitation possessed by the vital force, proceeding in accordance with the organic arrangement of the body, and not with deliberation of reason in overcoming an acute disease, is mostly a kind of allopathy. In order to relieve the primarily affected parts by a crisis, it frequently creates an increased and even tempestuous activity in the organs of secretion, for the purpose of transferring the disease from the former to the latter; the sequel is seen in the appearance of emesis, diarrhœa, flow of urine, perspiration, abscesses, etc., by which excitation of remote structures it is intended to establish a kind of derivation from originally morbid parts, because, under such circumstances, the nervous force dynamically excited, apparently strives to relieve its tension by the formation of material products.

It is only by the destruction and sacrifice of the system, that nature unassisted is enabled to rally from acute diseases, or slowly and imperfectly to re-establish health and harmony of life if death does not forestall her efforts.

After spontaneous recoveries, all this is pointed out by the great weakness and emaciation of the entire body, or of the parts having been affected by disease.

In a word, the whole process set up by the organism, in its self-limitation of diseases, exhibits to the observer nothing but suffering, and nothing that he could or should imitate if he truly exercises the art of healing.

[20] Daily experience shows the deplorable result obtained by this manœuvre in chronic diseases. *A cure is most rarely the result.* But who would call it a victory, when instead of attacking the enemy face to face, weapon to weapon, in order to destroy him and end with one blow his hostile incursions, he finds his cities sacked, his supplies cut off, his sustenance consumed, and everything devastated by fire and sword around him; by such measures the enemy may be obliged to give up in despair, but the object is not gained, the enemy is not crushed; he is still in the field, and when he has again obtained forage and supplies, he will lift his head with fiercer threats of vengeance; the enemy, I say, is by no means crushed, but the poor innocent country is so far ruined, that even time will scarcely restore its former condition. Such is allopathy in chronic diseases when it destroys the organism, without curing the disease, by its indirect attacks upon innocent parts, remote from the seat of disease. Such are its non-beneficent artifices!

[21] What good result was obtained by the frequent use of those artificial and offensive ulcers called fontanels? During the first few weeks, they really may have seemed slightly to check a chronic disorder by means of their antagonism, and as long as they continued to be painful, but as soon as the body had learned to bear them, they have never failed to weaken the patient, thereby increasing the range of the active chronic evil. It seems incredible that in the nineteenth cen-

tury it is thought possible that an opening could be made by such means for the escape of the *materia peccans.*

[22] Neither was a cure ever achieved by artificial evacuations.

[23] Such were the natural consequences of suppressing those local symptoms, consequences often represented by the allopathic physician as new and different diseases.

[24] Quite contrary to this method, the old school frequently ventures upon a directly opposite course, thus, by its repercussions and repellants, it would suppress at pleasure the efforts of vitality to relieve an inner disease, or troublesome local symptoms appearing on the surface of the body, by evacuants; it did not hesitate to treat chronic pains, sleeplessness, and inveterate diarrhœa with the most reckless doses of opium; or to suppress vomiting with effervescent saline mixtures, offensive perspiration of the feet by cold foot-baths, or preparations of lead or zinc; to counteract uterine hæmorrhage by injections of vinegar; colliquative sweats by alum whey; nocturnal seminal emissions by excessive use of camphor; frequent flushes of heat over the face or body by saltpetre, vegetable or sulphuric acid; to arrest nosebleed by closing the nares with plugs saturated with alcohol or astringent fluids, and to dry up with oxide of lead or zinc ichorous ulcers of the extremities, called forth by vital reaction to mitigate grave internal disease, etc.; but manifold experiences prove the lamentable consequences of such treatment.

By word and pen the old school practitioner boasts of being a rational physician, seeking for the cause of disease in order always to perform radical cures; but it is plain that his treatment is directed against a single symptom, always to the injury of the patient.

[25] A process termed enantiopathic with much propriety, to which allusion will be made in the text of the *Organon* (§ 59).

[26] Deafness was relieved only for a few hours by moderate shocks of the voltaic battery in the hands of the apothecary in fevers, but these soon ceased to be effective. In order to obtain other results, he was obliged to increase the power of the shocks until these too were unavailing. The strongest shocks at first improved the patient's hearing for a short time, but finally resulted in complete deafness

[27] Notwithstanding all this, Hufeland, the representative of the old school, exultingly praises these effects of digitalis (v. *Homœopathie,*

p. 22), in the following words, "No one can deny that violent excitement of circulation may be reduced by means of digitalis." An assertion entirely unsupported by experience.

[28] Supported in vain by Hufeland, in his pamphlet (*Die Homœopathie*, p. 20), for the sake of his inefficient practice (Unkunst).

Since allopathy, during twenty-five hundred years of its existence, remained ignorant of the source of most chronic diseases (psora), before the appearance of my book (*The Chronic Diseases*), it became necessary to invent a false explanation of the origin (genesis) of chronic disorders.

[29] *Quellan der Bisherigen Materia Medica.* Sources of the old Materia Medica preceding the third part of the "Pure Materia Medica."

[30] The absurdity of these drug mixtures has been recognized even by men of the prevailing school, although they followed this changeless routine in their own practice, and contrary to their own conviction. Thus Marcus Herz (in *Hufeland's Journ. der Pract.*, Arzt. ii, p. 33), expresses his conscientious scruples in the following words: "When we wish to relieve an inflammation, we do not use saltpetre, ammonia, or vegetable acids alone, but we often mix several, and frequently too many so-called antiphlogistic remedies together, or allow them to be used in rapid succession. When it becomes necessary to counteract putrefaction, we are not satisfied with the use of one well-known antiseptic, such as cinchona bark, mineral acids, arnica, or snake-root administered in large quantity, and to await the result; but we prefer to compound several of these drugs, and to count upon their united action; or from ignorance of the efficacy of any single drug in a given case, we huddle a variety of things together, and trust that by chance one of them may have the desired effect. Thus one remedy seldom is used to promote perspiration, to improve the blood (?), to liquefy accumulations (?), to produce expectoration or evacuation of the intestines; for such purposes our prescriptions are always complicated, never simple and pure, and *consequently we arrive at no definite or precise experiences regarding the effects of the individual ingredients of these prescriptions.* We have, nevertheless, arranged our remedies methodically according to their rank, and call that drug to which we ascribe the main action *basis;* we designate the rest as adjuvants, corrigents, etc. This classification is obviously an arbitrary one. Adjuvants take part in the total effect as well as the principal ingredient, although we have no means of determining the degree of their action; nor is the influence exercised by the corrigens upon the other drugs, a matter of indifference, since it must increase or decrease their action or give it another direction. We are therefore always bound to regard a cura-

tive (?) effect wrought by such a formula as the collective result of all its ingredients ; *nor can we obtain a clear idea of the separate action of each individual ingredient. In fact, our insight into that condition which determines an essential knowledge of all our remedies, as well as our knowledge of the manifold relationships into which they enter when mixed together, is far too imperfect to allow us to determine the magnitude and variety of the effects of a drug, however insignificant it may appear if introduced into the human body combined with other substances.*

[31] For truth is of the same eternal origin as the omniscient and beneficent Divinity. Men may leave it long unheeded until its rays of light penetrate with irresistible force the mist of prejudices, like the dawn of approaching day, that shall shine brightly and forever for the welfare of mankind.

[32] Examples of this kind may be found in the preceding editions of the *Organon of the Healing Art.*

[33] It was the usual practice to attempt to promote arrested cutaneous excretions, by prescribing an infusion of elder flowers, to be drank during the chills of a fever occasioned by exposure. This infusion by virtue of its similarity of action (homœopathic), may cure the fever, and restore the patient quickly, and much more successfully without perspiration if taken by itself. Hard and acute swellings, the excessive and painful inflammation of which prevents transition into suppuration, were usually covered by repeated hot poultices, and behold, inflammation and pain were speedily diminished by the formation of the abscess, indicated by a yellowish shining prominence and fluctuation. The hardness was then supposed to have been softened by the moisture of the poultice, while actually the higher temperature of the latter had relieved homœopathically the excess of inflammation, thus facilitating the formation of the abscess. Why is the red oxide of mercury, which is known to produce inflammation of the eyes, employed with benefit in some kinds of ophthalmia, in the form of St. Yves salve? Is it so difficult to recognize the homœopathic nature of this process? Or, why should a little juice of parsley bring instantaneous relief in cases of strangury, common among young children, or in cases of clap, chiefly marked by frequent and ineffectual efforts to urinate, if this freshly prepared juice did not produce by itself, in healthy persons, that painful and ineffectual straining, which proves the homœopathic nature of its curative effect.

Pimpernel root, increasing the mucous secretion of the air-passages and fauces, was effectually used in curing the so-called mucous cramp (bronchial catarrh).

The leaves of the Sabina, themselves capable of producing uterine hæmorrhage, were used successfully in such cases, without, however, leading to the recognition of the homœopathic law of cure. In cases of strangulated hernia and ileus, many physicians found a superior and reliable remedy in small doses of opium, which has the property of checking intestinal evacuations; notwithstanding this circumstance, they did not perceive the operation of the homœopathic law in such cases. They cured non-venereal ulcers of the throat with small doses of mercury, homœopathic to these cases; they frequently checked diarrhœa with small doses of cathartic rhubarb; they cured hydrophobia with Belladonna, capable of producing a similar affection, and removed as if by magic the dangerous comatose condition of inflammatory fevers with a small dose of opium, known to be heating and stupefying. And yet they vituperate homœopathy, and persecute it with a degree of wrath that can only be excited in an incorrigible heart by the admonitions of an evil conscience.

[34] From these examples, derived from domestic practice, Mr. M. Lux has constructed his so-called curative method according to *equals* and *Idem*, called by him *Isopathy*, which some eccentric minds have already declared as the *non plus ultra* of curative methods, without knowing how it could be realized.

If these examples are carefully considered, the matter will appear in a very different light.

The purely physical forces are of different nature from dynamic medicinal powers in their effect upon the living organism.

The degree of warmth or cold of the surrounding atmosphere, of water, or of food and drink, do not (considered as *warmth* or *cold*) *per se*, condition an absolute hurtfulness for the healthy body; warmth and cold in their changes are necessary for the maintenance of health, consequently they are not medicines *per se;* warmth and cold therefore applied to bodily affections do not act as remedial agents by virtue of their nature (not as warmth and cold considered as hurtful things, *per se*, in the manner of drugs, like rhubarb, bark, etc., even if reduced to the finest doses), but only by virtue of their greater or smaller quantity, *i. e.*, according to the degree of their temperature; thus (to use an example of mere physical forces), a large leaden weight would press the hand painfully, not by virtue of its being lead, but by means of its quantity and heaviness in a mass, while a thin leaden plate would cause no suffering.

If warmth and cold therefore are beneficial in burns and freezing, they are so on account of their degree of temperature, in the same manner as their extremes of temperature are obnoxious to the healthy body.

Accordingly we find that, in these examples of domestic practice, the frozen limb is not restored by the continued degree of cold applied to it (because that would have benumbed and killed it); but it is by a degree of cold (homœopathy) which is gradually reduced to a comfortable temperature approaching that of the limb. Thus, frozen cabbage applied to the frozen hand in the temperature of the room will soon melt, and by gradually rising from a temperature of + 1 to 2, and so on to that of the room, say + 10°, becoming gradually warmer, will thus restore the limb homœopathically. Neither is a hand scalded by boiling water, restored according to the principle of *isopathy* by the application of boiling water, but only by a lower degree of heat. For instance, if the hand is held in a vessel containing a fluid heated to 60°, this will grow cooler every minute, gradually assuming the temperature of the room; thus the burned part will have been cured *homœopathically*. The first cannot be drawn *isopathically* from potatoes or apples by means of water, which is rapidly becoming ice, but only by water remaining near the freezing-point.

Thus, to use another illustration of physical effects: the suffering occasioned by a blow upon the forehead by some hard body (of a severe bruise), is soon lessened by pressing the thumb hard upon the place for a while, gradually diminishing the pressure: this is homœopathic relief; while an equally severe blow upon the sore place, with an equally hard body, would be isopathy; but it would increase the evil.

The same book contains further examples of isopathic cures, such as muscular contractions in the human body and spinal paralysis in a dog, both caused by cold, and rapidly cured by cold bathing. This circumstance is erroneously explained as being the result of isopathy. Disorders resulting from cold have merely the name of colds, but are frequently occasioned in a predisposed person by a breath of wind which was not even cold. Neither can the various effects of a cold bath upon the living body of well or sick persons, be embraced so completely in one principle, that a system could so boldly be at once built upon it. That snake-bites, as there stated, are positively cured by parts of snakes, would be counted among the fables of bygone ages, until such improbable assertions have been established by undoubted observations and experiences, an event scarcely to be looked for. Finally, it is said that the saliva of a rabid dog, given to a man (in Russia), raving with hydrophobia, cured him. It is to be hoped that such assertions, founded on hearsay, will mislead no conscientious physician to imitate so dangerous an experiment, or to build upon it a so-called system of isopathy, as dangerous as it is absurd in its extended sense, notwithstanding the praises of eccentric enthusiasts (though not of the modest author of the pamphlet entitled, *Isopathy of Contagions*, Leipsic, published by Kollmann), particularly Dr. Gross (*Allg. Hom. Z.*, ii, p. 72), who proclaims this isopathy (*æqualia æqualibus*) as the only true principle, while he considers *similia similibus* merely as makeshift. This is truly ungrateful, since he is indebted to *similia similibus* for reputation and fortune.

[35] Fernelius already (*Therap.*, lib. vi, cap. 20) considered the approximation of a burnt part to the fire as the appropriate remedy for the relief of pain. John Hunter (*On the Blood, Inflammation, etc.*, p. 218) alludes to the great disadvantage of treating burns with cold water, and gives decided preference to the approximation of fire, not according to transmitted medical doctrines, demanding (*contraria contrariis*) cooling applications for inflammations, but in harmony with the experience, that a similar application of heat is more beneficial (*similia similibus*).

[36] Sydenham (Opera, p. 271) says: "*Alcohol*, frequently applied, is preferable to any other remedy in burns." Also Benjamin Bell (*System of Surgery*, 3d edit., 1789), pays homage to experience, which shows homœopathic remedies to be the only beneficial ones. He says: "One of the best remedies for burns is *alcohol*. During its application it appears to increase the pain for a moment (§ 164), but this soon subsides, leaving an agreeable, quieting sensation. It acts most potently when the parts are immersed in the alcohol; where that cannot be done, the parts must continually be covered by pieces of linen moistened with alcohol." But I must add: *The warm, and even very warm alcohol brings more rapid and more certain relief in these cases, because it is much more homœopathic than if unwarmed.* And this is abundantly confirmed by experience.

[37] Edward Kentish, who treated the frightful burns of workmen in the coal-mines, occasioned by inflammable vapors, orders "the application of heated oil of turpentine, or alcohol, as the most excellent remedy in extensive and severe burns." (*Essay on Burns*, London, 1798, second essay.) No treatment can be more homœopathic than this, neither is there a more beneficial one.

The honest and highly experienced Heister (*Institut. Chirurg.*, tom. i, p. 333) confirms this by his experience, and praises "the application of oil of turpentine, alcohol, and hot poultices, as *hot* as they can be borne."

These (homœopathic) remedies, capable of producing by themselves burning sensations and heat, undeniably show their wonderful superiority over the cooling and cold remedies, if applied to parts inflamed by a burn; provided, however, the experiment is properly conducted in such a manner that both curative methods are, for the sake of comparison, applied to the same person, suffering from burns of equal degrees of severity.

Thus, John Bell (S. Kühn's *Phys. Med. Journal*, Leipsic, 1801, June,

p. 428), had one arm of a scalded woman moistened with *oil of turpentine*, while the other was immersed *in cold water*. The first arm was well in half an hour, but the latter continued to be painful for six hours. If withdrawn from the water only for a moment, *the patient experienced far greater pain, requiring far more time for relief than the arm treated with turpentine.*

John Anderson (Kentish, *loc. cit.* p. 43) treated a woman who had burned her face and arm with boiling fat. "The face, which was much burned and red, and very painful, was covered in a few minutes with oil of turpentine, but she had voluntarily placed her arm in cold water, desiring to treat it in that way for a few hours. In seven hours her face already looked much better, and was relieved. She had often repeated the applications of cold water to the arm, but when she omitted them she complained of much pain; in fact the inflammation was found to have *increased*. On the following morning I found that she had suffered much pain in the arm during the night; the inflammation extended above the elbow; various large blisters had opened, and thick crusts had formed upon the arm and hand, to which a warm poultice was now applied. But the face was completely painless; the arm, on the contrary, had to be dressed for a fortnight with emollients, before it healed."

Who would not recognize in these cases the great superiority of the (HOMŒOPATHIC) *treatment, by remedies of similar effect, over the inferior treatment by contraries* (CONTRARIA CONTRARIIS), *according to antiquated rules of common practice.*

[38] Not only John Hunter (*loc. cit.*) alludes to the great disadvantages of treating burns with cold water, but also W. Fabric. von Hilden (*De combustionibus libellus*, Basil, 1607, cap. 5, p. 11), says: "Cold applications are very injurious in burns, and produce the most evil consequences, such as inflammation, suppuration, and sometimes gangrene."

[39] Zimmermann (*Über die Erfahrung*, ii, p. 318), informs us that the inhabitants of hot countries successfully resort to that practice, taking some spirituous liquor when they become excessively heated.

[40] The following quotations from authors, having a presentiment of homœopathy, are not brought forward for the purpose of proving the stability of this doctrine, sufficiently firm in itself, but they are introduced to escape the accusation of having ignored those presentiments, for the sake of the credit of securing the priority of the idea.

[41] Basil, *Froben*, 1538, § 72.

[42] *Mémoirs de l'Académie Royale*, 1710.

[43] *Eph. Nat. Cur. Cent.*, X, obs. 76.

[44] *Medicin. Electrisität*, II, pp. 15 and 282.

[45] *Mémoire lu à l'Acad. de Caen.*

[46] *Libell. de stram*, p. 8.

[47] Jo. Hummellii, *Commentatio de arthritide tam tartarea, quam scorbutica, seu podagra et scorbuto.* Büdingae, 1738, 8, pp. 40–42.

ORGANON OF THE ART OF HEALING.

§ 1. THE physician's highest and *only* calling is to restore health to the sick, which is called Healing.[1]

§ 2. The highest aim of healing is the speedy, gentle, and permanent restitution of health, or alleviation and obliteration of disease in its entire extent, in the shortest, most reliable, and safest manner, according to clearly intelligible reasons.

§ 3. The physician should distinctly understand the following conditions: what is curable in diseases in general, and in each individual case in particular; that is, the recognition of disease (*indicatio*). He should clearly comprehend what is curative in drugs in general, and in each drug in particular; that is, he should possess a perfect knowledge of medicinal powers. He should be governed by distinct reasons, in order to insure recovery, by adapting what is curative in medicines to what he has recognized as undoubtedly morbid in a patient; that is to say, he should adapt it so that the case is met by a remedy well matched with regard to its kind of action (selection of the remedy, *indicatum*), its necessary preparation and quantity (proper dose), and the proper time of its repetition. Finally, when the physician knows in each case the obstacles in the way of recovery, and how to remove them, he is prepared to act thoroughly, and to the purpose, as a true master of the art of healing.

§ 4. He is at the same time a preserver of health when he knows the causes that disturb health, that produce and maintain disease, and when he knows how to remove them from healthy persons.

§ 5. The physician in curing derives assistance from the knowledge of facts concerning the most *probable cause* of acute disease, as well as from the most significant points in the entire history of a case of chronic disease; aided by such knowledge, he is enabled to discover the *primary cause* of the latter, dependent mostly on a chronic miasm. In connection with this, the bodily constitution of a patient (particularly if he has a chronic disease), the character of his mind and temperament, his occupation, his mode of living and habits, his social and domestic relations, his age and sexual function, etc., are to be taken into consideration.

§ 6. An unbiassed observer, though of unequalled sagacity, impressed with the futility of transcendental speculation unsupported by experience, observes in each individual disease only what is outwardly discernible through the senses, viz., changes in the sensorial condition (health) of body and soul—*morbid signs or symptoms.* In other words, he observes deviations from the previous healthy condition of the patient, felt by him, and recognized upon him by his attendants, and observed upon him by the physician. All of these observable signs together represent the disease in its full extent; that is, they constitute together the true and only conceivable form of the disease.[2]

§ 7. In a disease presenting no manifest exciting or maintaining cause (*causa occasionalis*) for removal,[3] nothing is to be discerned but symptoms. These alone (with due regard to the possible existence of some miasm, and to accessory circumstances, § 5) must constitute the medium through which the disease demands and points out its curative agent. Hence the totality of these symptoms, *this outwardly reflected image of the inner nature of the disease, i. e., of the suffering vital force*, must be the chief or only means of the disease to make known the remedy necessary for its cure, the only means of determining the selection of the appropriate remedial agent. In short, the totality of the symptoms must be regarded by the physician as the principal and only condition to be recognized and removed by his art in each case of disease, that it may be cured and converted into health.[4]

§ 8. It is as impossible to conceive as to demonstrate by human experience that, after the removal of every symptom of a disease embraced in the totality of perceptible phenomena, anything but health should or possibly could remain, or, that after such removal, the morbid process of the interior could still continue to be active.[5]

§ 9. During the healthy condition of man this spirit-like force (autocracy), animating the material body (organism), rules supreme as *dynamis*. By it all parts are maintained wonderfully in harmonious vital process, both in feelings and functions, in order that our intelligent mind may be free to make the living, healthy, bodily medium subservient to the higher purpose of our being.

§ 10. The material organism without vital force is incapable[6] of feeling activity or self-preservation. This immaterial being (vital force) alone, animating the organism in the state of sickness and of health, imparts the faculty of feeling, and controls the functions of life.

§ 11. In sickness this spirit-like, self-acting (automatic) vital force, omnipresent in the organism, is alone primarily deranged by the dynamic influence of some morbific agency inimical to life. Only this abnormally modified vital force can excite morbid sensations in the organism, and determine the abnormal functional activity which we call disease. This force, itself invisible, becomes perceptible only through its effects upon the organism, makes known, and has no other way of making known its morbid disturbance to the observer and physician than by the manifestation of morbid feelings and functions; that is, *by symptoms of disease* in the visible material organism.

§ 12. Diseases are produced only by the morbidly disturbed vital force,[7] hence the manifestations of disease discernible by our senses, at the same time represent every internal change (*i. e.*, the entire morbid disturbance of the dynamis), and expose to view, so to speak, the whole disease. It follows that after the cure of such manifestations of disease, and of all discoverable aberrations from healthy vital functions, their disappearance must necessarily and with equal certainty be presumed to result in, and to determine the restoration of the integrity of vital force, and the return of health to the entire organism.

§ 13. Hence, disease (not subject to the manual skill of surgery), considered by allopathists as a material thing hidden within, but distinct from the living whole (the organism and its lifegiving vital force), is a nonentity, however subtile it is thought to be. It could have originated only in the minds of materialists, and has for thousands of years imparted to medical science manifold deplorable directions, stamping it as an unwholesome instead of a healing art.

§ 14. Within the human body there is no curable disorder, nor any curable invisible morbid change, that does not make itself known as disease to the exact observer by means of signs and symptoms, quite in accordance with the infinite goodness of divine Wisdom.

§ 15. Hence the affection of that morbidly altered, spirit-like dynamis (vital force) animating our body, and residing unseen in its interior, and the complex of externally perceptible symptoms caused by that power in the organism, and representing the actual disease, constitute a whole—one and the same. Although the organism as material instrument serves for the purpose of life, still this organism is as inconceivable without animation derived from the instinctive feeling and controlling vital force, as the vital force without the organism; consequently both constitute a unit, although our reason in its process of thought separates this unit into two ideas for the convenience of comprehension.

§ 16. Our vital force, that spirit-like dynamis, cannot be reached nor affected except by a spirit-like (dynamic) process, resulting from the hurtful influences of hostile agencies from the outer world acting upon the healthy organism, and disturbing the harmonious process of life. Neither can the physician free the vital force from any of these morbid disturbances, *i. e.*, diseases, except likewise by spirit-like (dynamic, virtual) alterative powers of the appropriate remedies acting upon our spirit-like vital force, perceiving this remedial power through the omnipresent susceptibility of the nerves of the organism. Thus, healing remedies can and actually do restore health and vital harmony only by virtue of their dynamic action upon the vital force, after those changes in the health of the patient (totality of symptoms), perceivable by our senses, have represented the disease to the attentively observing physician, as completely as possible for the purpose of its cure.

§ 17. In effecting a cure, the inner change of vital force, forming the basis of disease, that is the totality of disease, is always cancelled[8] by removing the entire complex of perceptible signs and disturbances of the disease. Hence it follows that the physician has only to remove the entire complex of symptoms, in order to cancel and obliterate[9] simultaneously the internal change; that is, the morbidly altered vital force, the totality of the disease, in fact, the *disease itself.* But disease obliterated is health restored, the highest and only object of the physician impressed with the significance of his calling, which does not consist in the use of learned phrases, but in bringing relief.

§ 18. It is then unquestionably true that, besides the totality of symptoms, it is impossible to discover any other manifestation by which diseases could express their need of relief. Hence it undeniably follows that the totality of symptoms observed in each individual case of disease, can be the *only indication* to guide us in the selection of a remedy.

§ 19. Now since *diseases* are definable only as *aberra-*

tions from the state of health, which declare themselves by symptoms, and since a cure also becomes possible only by *changing this aberration of feeling back into the healthy state*, we may readily understand how impossible it would be to cure diseases by *medicines* unless these possessed the power of altering* the state of health dependent on feelings and functions of the organism. In fact, the curative power of medicines must rest *alone* on their power of altering the sensorial condition of the body.

§ 20. Neither the spirit-like power concealed in drugs, and shown by their ability of altering the health of man, nor their power of curing diseases, can be comprehended by a mere effort of reason; it is only through manifestations of their effect upon the state of health that this power of drugs is experienced and distinctly observed.

§ 21. It is then undeniable that the healing property of drugs is actually undiscernible in itself, and that even the purest experiments, conducted by the most actute observer, fail to reveal any peculiarities of drugs, marking them at once as medicines or healing remedies. It is possible only to recognize the power of drugs to produce distinct changes in the state of feeling of the human body, particularly of the *healthy human body*, and to excite numerous definite morbid symptoms in and about the same; and it follows that, if drugs act as curative remedies, they exercise this curative power only by virtue of their faculty of altering bodily feelings through the production of peculiar symptoms. Consequently those morbid disturbances, called forth by drugs in the healthy

* *Umstimmen* means literally to alter the pitch; to retune.

body, must be accepted as the only possible revelation of their inherent curative power. Through them only we are able to discover what capacity of producing disease, and hence, also, what capacity of curing disease is possessed by each individual drug.

§ 22. Hence there is no discoverable part that can be removed from a disease for the purpose of restoring health, except the totality of its signs and symptoms. Hence, also, drugs manifest no other curative power except their tendency to produce morbid symptoms in healthy persons, and to remove them from the sick. Thus it follows, on the one hand, that drugs become curative remedies capable of obliterating disease only through their power of creating certain disturbances and symptoms; that is, by producing a certain artificial diseased condition, they cancel and exterminate the symptoms already present, *i. e.*, the natural diseased condition which it is intended to cure. It follows, however, on the other hand, that a remedy must be found for the totality of symptoms of the disease to be cured, which remedy is inclined to produce either similar or contrary symptoms, according to the dictates of experience, which must prove either similar or contrary drug-symptoms[10] to be most serviceable with regard to ease, certainty, and permanency in cancelling or converting into health the symptoms of disease.

§ 23. Each real experience, and exact experiment will convince us that persistent symptoms of disease are so imperfectly alleviated or exterminated by *contrary* symptoms of a drug (used according to *antipathic, enantiopathic*, or *palliative* method), that after a brief period of apparent relief they will break forth again in a more marked degree, and visibly aggravated. (See §§ 58–62 and 69.)

§ 24. So there remains no other manner of applying drugs in the cure of diseases but the homœopathic method, in accordance with which we select a drug to meet the totality of symptoms of the case of disease, which drug should possess the power and inclination in a higher degree than any other (of all drugs known and proved with regard to their tendency to alter the feelings of a healthy person), of producing an artificial morbid condition most similar to that of the natural disease.

§ 25. But now actual experience,[11] the only infallible oracle of medical art, teaches in every carefully conducted experiment that *that* drug, proved in its effect upon healthy persons, to produce the greatest number of symptoms similar to those found in a case of disease to be cured, and when administered in properly potentiated* and diminished doses, will rapidly, thoroughly, and permanently cancel and turn into health the totality of symptoms of this diseased condition; that is (see §§ 6–16), the entire present case of disease. Experience also teaches that all drugs will unexceptionally cure diseases, the symptoms of which are as similar as possible to those of the drugs, and leave none uncured.

§ 26. This is based upon that homœopathic law of nature which, hitherto unacknowledged, though not unrecognized, had even been the foundation of every real cure. In the living organism *a weaker dynamic affection is permanently extinguished by a stronger one if the*

---

* Potentized.

latter (deviating in kind) is very similar in its manifestation to the former.[12]

§ 27. Therefore, the healing power of medicines rests upon their faculty of producing symptoms similar to the disease, and superior to it in strength (§§ 12–26), so that each individual case of disease is most certainly, fundamentally, and rapidly extinguished and cancelled by a drug which is more potent than the disease, and capable of producing in the body symptoms most similar to, and completely resembling the totality of those of the disease.

§ 28. Since this natural law of cure has been verified to the world by every pure experiment and genuine experience, and has thus become an established fact, a scientific explanation of *its mode of action* is of little importance; I therefore place but a slight value upon an attempt at explanation. Nevertheless, the following view holds good as the most probable one, since it is based entirely upon empirical premises.

§ 29. We have seen *that every disease (not subject to surgery alone) is based upon some particular morbid derangement in the feelings and functions of the vital force; and thus, in the process of a homœopathic cure, by administering a medicinal potency chosen exactly in accordance with the similitude of symptoms, a somewhat stronger, similar, artificial morbid affection is implanted upon the vital power deranged by a natural disease; this artificial affection is substituted, as it were, for the weaker similar natural disease (morbid excitation), against which the instinctive vital force, now only excited to stronger effort* *by the drug-affection,* needs only to direct its increased energy; but owing to its brief duration*[13] *it will soon be overcome by the vital force, which, liberated first from the natural disease, and finally from the substituted artificial (drug-) affection, now again finds itself enabled to continue the life of the organism in health.* This very probable process is based upon the following propositions:

§ 30. Natural diseases are cured and overcome by proper medicines, because the health of the human body seems to be more readily affected by drugs (also because it is in our power to regulate their dose) than by natural morbific agencies.

§ 31. Those partly psychical and partly physical terrestrial potencies known as noxious influences, inimical to life, do not possess the morbific power of modifying[14] human health unconditionally; but they produce sickness only at a time when our organism happens to be sufficiently disposed and inclined to become affected, and to have its feeling of health altered into morbidly abnormal sensations and functions by the morbific cause that is present. These potencies, therefore, do not make every one sick, nor can they do so at all times.

§ 32. The case is far different with artificial, morbific potencies which we call medicines. For every true

---

* The words of the text are: "*Die instinctartige Lebenskraft, nun bloss noch (aber stärker) arzneikrank.*" Translated literally, this reads: "*The instinctive vital force, now only (stronger) diseased by the drug affection*" Although this defines the process, it does not render it as intelligible to the student as the slight modification: "*Now only excited to stronger effort,*" etc. —TRANSLATOR.

medicine (drug) acts at all times, and under *all* circumstances, upon *every* living human being, and excites its peculiar symptoms in the organism (even very perceptibly if the dose is large enough). Thus, every living human organism is always (*unconditionally*) affected, and, as it were, infected by the drug disease which, as stated, is not at all the case with natural diseases.

§ 33. Consequently, experience[15] leads to the undeniable conclusion that the living, human organism is far more disposed and inclined to be affected, and to have its feelings altered by medicinal powers than by other noxious agencies and contagious miasms; or, to express the same in other words: *extraneous, noxious agencies possess a subordinate, and often extremely conditional power; but drug potencies possess an absolute, unconditional power, far superior to the former in its* ability to produce ill health (morbid discordancy) of the human body.

§ 34. The greater intensity of artificial diseases produced by drugs, does not constitute the only condition of their ability to cure natural diseases. In order to perform a cure, it is necessary that drugs should possess the power of producing in the human body an artificial disease, *most similar to that which is to be cured;* for it is by virtue of its similitude, combined with greater intensity, that the drug disease is substituted for the natural disease, thus depriving the latter of its power to affect the vital force. This is true to such an extent, that even nature herself is unable to cure an older disease through the accession of a new, *dissimilar* affection, even of great intensity; nor can the physician perform a cure by means of drugs *incapable of producing in the organism a diseased condition similar to that which is to be cured.*

§ 35. In order to illustrate the preceding, let us examine three different instances of the process adopted by nature when two unlike natural diseases meet in the human body, and then let us consider the result of the ordinary allopathic treatment of diseases with improper medicines which are incapable of producing an artificial morbid condition similar to that which is to be cured; it will then become apparent that nature herself is unable to extinguish a given dissimilar disease by means of an unhomœopathic, though stronger, affection; and that the most powerful drugs, if not homœopathic, will be unable to cure any disease whatever.

§ 36. I. Two *dissimilar* diseases coexisting in the human body may be of equal intensity; or, in case the *older one* of the two proves to be of the greater *intensity*, then the new disease is kept away and excluded from the body. Thus, a patient already afflicted with an intractable chronic disease, will not be attacked by moderate autumnal dysentery, or any other epidemic. According to Larry,[16] the Levantine plague does not visit localities where scurvy prevails; neither does it attack persons suffering from herpes. According to Jenner, vaccination proves abortive in persons suffering from rickets. Von Hildebrand says that patients in the ulcerative stages of consumption, are not infected by fevers of a mild epidemic form.

§ 37. And thus, an old chronic disease will remain stationary and uncured under the *ordinary allopathic treatment* even if persisted in for years, that is, if the case had not been too harshly treated with drugs that, by themselves, cannot produce in healthy persons a condition similar to the disease. Examples of this kind may be observed in daily practice, and therefore require no further illustration.

§ 38. II. Or, the *new dissimilar disease may be of greater intensity.* In that case, the first disease affecting the patient, being the weaker, will be postponed and suspended by the superadded intenser malady until the latter has terminated its course, or has been cured; whereupon the old disease will reappear *uncured.* Thus Tulpius[17] informs us that two children, affected by a species of epilepsy, were at once free from that disease, when they were attacked by *tinea capitis;* but as soon as the eruption disappeared from the head, the epilepsy returned in the same manner as before. It was observed by Schöpf[18] that the itch disappeared when scurvy attacked the patient; but came to light again after the scurvy was cured. In the same manner, the suppurative stage of consumption became suspended upon the accession of violent typhus fever; but continued its progress when the fever had ceased.[19] Whenever insanity is combined with consumption, the latter, with all its symptoms, is suspended by the former; but as soon as the insanity subsides, consumption returns at once to end the life of the patient.[20] When measles and small-pox prevail at the same time, and both infect the same child, the measles are usually arrested in their course by the eruption of small-pox appearing somewhat later; but again resume their progress when the small-pox has disappeared. Nevertheless, it frequently happened that small-pox, breaking forth after inoculation, was arrested during four days by the eruption of measles occurring meanwhile; after desquamation of the measles, the small-pox was seen to run its course to its end, as observed by Manget.[21] Also measles, breaking out on the sixth day after the effectual inoculation of small-pox, have been known to arrest the inflammation caused by the inoculation of that virus, so that the variola-pustules did not appear until the measles had terminated their course of seven days.[22] On the fourth or fifth day after inoculation of small-pox, during the prevalence of an epidemic of measles, in many persons the measles prevented the eruption of small-pox until the former had completed their course; thereupon the variola appeared, and terminated favorably.[23] The genuine, smooth, erysipelatous scarlatina of Sydenham,[24] complicated with angina faucium, has been arrested on the fourth day by the eruption of vaccine-pustules, after the termination of which, the scarlatina returned. As both diseases appear to be of equal intensity, an eruption of cow-pox was suspended in the same manner on the eighth day by the accession of genuine, smooth scarlet fever of Sydenham; and the red areola of the former was seen to subside until the scarlet fever had ended, when the vaccine-pustule progressed to its termination.[25] In the other instance observed by Kortum,[26] cow-pox was suspended by measles: on the eighth day, when the cow-pox approached its perfection, measles broke out; the cow-pox now came to a stand, and did not terminate its course until after desquamation of the measles, so that the cow-pox appeared on the sixteenth day as it usually does on the tenth. The same author testifies[27] that, even during the presence of the eruption of measles, vaccination proved effectual, but did not run its course until the measles had ended theirs.

I myself saw a case of mumps (*angina parotidea*) vanish when, after vaccination, the cow-pox was approaching its perfection; and not until it had completely terminated its course, and the red areolæ had disappeared, did that febrile swelling of the parotid and submaxillary glands return again by virtue of its peculiar miasm, progressing through its period of seven days.

Thus, whenever two dissimilar diseases meet in the body, the stronger one always suspends the weaker (provided they do not combine, which seldom happens in the acute forms); *but they never cure each other.*

§ 39. For hundreds of years this state of things was witnessed with indifference by the ordinary school of medicine; it saw that not even nature could cure any disease by superadding another, however intense, if the latter was *dissimilar* to the one already present in the body. In the presence of such facts, it was reprehensible on the part of that school to persist in treating chronic diseases allopathically; that is, with medicines and recipes capable of producing every variety of morbid effects, almost invariably *dissimilar* to those of the disease to be cured. And, though physicians had hitherto neglected to observe nature correctly, the deplorable results of their treatment should have led them to conclude that their means were ill-adapted to the purpose, and their course a wrong one. They should have known that, while they were directing severe allopathic treatment (as was commonly the case) against a chronic disease, they were merely creating an artificial disease *dissimilar* to the original one; this, while it was kept up, only quieted, suppressed, and suspended the original malady, always breaking forth again, as a matter of course, whenever the decline of the patient's strength no longer permitted the continuance of these allopathic measures. It is true that frequently repeated purgatives will shortly cause the eruption of itch to disappear from the skin; but when the patient ceases to endure the (dissimilar) intestinal disease forced upon him, and when he can no longer swallow those purgatives, the cutaneous eruption either reappears in its former shape, or the internal psora is developed into some threatening symptom, burdening the patient with painfully deranged digestion and debility in addition to his undiminished original evil. Thus, when ordinary practitioners keep up artificial, cutaneous ulcers and fontanels upon the surface of the body, in order to exterminate some chronic disease, they can *never* gain their object, nor cure the disease in that manner, because such artificial, cutaneous ulcers are entirely foreign and allopathic to the internal disease. It is only now and then rendered dormant, and suspended for a few weeks, when the irritation created by severe fontanels happens to be a more intense (dissimilar) disorder than the internal disease; but it is mere temporary suspension while the patient's health declines. Pechlin[28] and others assert that epilepsy, suppressed for many years by means of fontanels, invariably returns in an aggravated form when the issues are allowed to heal. If purgatives and issues are dissimilar, allopathic, and debilitating remedies in itch and epilepsy, it is impossible to conceive of treatment more inappropriate than that by means of recipes, only too commonly compounded of unknown ingredients, and employed in ordinary practice in nameless and countless other forms of disease. These mixtures are also weakening by suppressing and suspending the evils only for a short time without curing them, while their protracted use always adds a new, morbid condition on the old one.

§ 40. III. *The new disease*, after exerting its influence for a long time upon the organism, may join the *old, dissimilar malady*, forming with the latter a *complicated* evil. Each disorder occupies a certain region of the organism; that is, each chooses, as it were, the most accessible organs and locality most peculiarly suited to it, while it leaves the remaining territory in possession of the other, dissimilar disease. Thus a person afflicted with syphilis, may, in addition, be affected by the itch, and *vice versâ. As two dissimilar diseases, they cannot obliterate or cure each other.* The syphilitic symptoms at first remain dormant and suspended, while the itch eruption begins to appear; but in due course of time, the venereal disease being at least of equal intensity with the itch, they are associated;[29] that is, each occupies those portions of the organism most adapted to it; but the condition of the patient is thereby seriously aggravated, and far more difficult to cure.

When dissimilar, acute, contagious diseases, for instance small-pox and measles, meet in the body, they generally suspend each other, as before remarked; but there have been violent epidemics of this kind presenting the rare phenomenon of two dissimilar, acute diseases simultaneously attacking one person, thus forming a complication for a short time. During an epidemic where small-pox and measles prevailed at the same time, these diseases either avoided or suspended each other; the measles did not appear until twenty days after the small-pox eruption, while the latter did not attack persons until the seventeenth or eighteenth day after the appearance of the measles, so that the first disease had ample time to complete its course. Among 300 of such cases, there was but one in which P. Russel[30] recognized both dissimilar diseases at the same time upon one person. Rainey[31] twice observed small-pox and measles together in the case of two girls. J. Maurice[32] declares that he has seen in his whole practice only two such cases. Statements of this kind are made by Ettmüller[33] and others.

Cow-pox was observed by Zenker[34] to run its regular course by the side of purple rash and measles; and Jenner made the same observation during a course of mercurial treatment in a case of syphilis.

§ 41. In ordinary practice, such complicated diseases, produced by inappropriate treatment (allopathic method of cure), and prolonged use of ill-adapted medicines, are by far more frequent than natural diseases, associated and complicated with each other in one organism. Through the influence of a frequently repeated and inappropriate medicine, possessing peculiar powers of its own, new and often very protracted morbid conditions are associated with the natural disease, instead of curing it. These new morbid conditions are gradually blended and complicated with the dissimilar, chronic malady which they were unable to cure homœopathically by similitude of effect; they add to the old disease a new, dissimilar, artificial one of chronic character, thus doubling the hitherto simple case, which thus becomes far more severe and intractable, nay, often quite incurable. These statements are corroborated by numerous cases reported in medical journals and treatises. There are numerous cases of this kind where venereal chancre, complicated with itch-disease, or also with the dyscrasia of sycotic gonorrhœa (Feigwarzentripper), remains uncured by protracted and inappropriate treatment with large and frequent doses of mercurials, and where it becomes complicated with chronic, mercurial disease,[35] gradually generated in the organism. Thus, a monstrous complication is formed, known by the general term of masked syphilis, which, if not entirely incurable, is most difficult to eradicate.

§ 42. Nature herself, as above stated, in some instances

permits the combination of two (or even of three) natural diseases in the same body. But it should be well understood that such a complication can only be entered into by diseases *dissimilar to each other;* and which, according to eternal laws of nature, can neither neutralize, annihilate, nor cure each other; whence it appears as if both (or the three), so to speak, divided the organism between them, and that each occupied those parts of the system best adapted to it. The dissimilarity of these diseases renders such a combination possible.

§ 43. But the result is far different, when two similar diseases meet in the organism; that is, when a stronger and similar disease is added to the one already present. A case of this kind demonstrates how nature may accomplish cures, and how this object should be achieved by human skill.

§ 44. Two diseases *similar* in character cannot, like dissimilar diseases (in instance I), *repel* one another; nor can they, like dissimilar diseases (in instance II), *suspend* each other, so that the older could return after the termination of the more recent disease; nor can two *similar* diseases, like dissimilar affections (as in example III), exist *side by side*, or form a *double*, complicated disease in the organism.

§ 45. On the contrary, two diseases, though different in kind,[36] but very similar in regard to their manifestation of suffering and symptoms, will always extinguish each other whenever they meet in the organism; the stronger disease will overcome the weaker one, for reasons not difficult to divine: the superadded stronger morbific potency, on account of its similitude of effect, takes possession chiefly of *the same parts* in the organism hitherto affected by the weaker, morbific agency; this is thereby deprived of its power of action, and is consequently extinguished[37]. In other words, as soon as the vital force, disturbed by the morbific potency hitherto acting upon it, is more powerfully affected by the new and most similar (but stronger, dynamic) morbific potency, the latter continues *alone* to affect the vital force; and in this manner the former similar, but weaker agency, being a mere dynamic power without substance, must consequently cease to exist, and hence, cease to exert its morbific influence upon the vital force.

§ 46. Many examples might be enumerated where, in the course of nature, diseases were homœopathically cured by others of similar symptoms. But in order to furnish definite and real instances, it will be necessary to choose a limited class of diseases which, arising from a fixed miasm, are always uniform and known by a definite name. Prominent among them is variola, dreaded on account of the large number of its violent symptoms, and known to have obliterated and cured numerous evils by means of the similitude of its symptoms. It is, for example, common during small-pox to meet with violent forms of ophthalmia, often ending in blindness; and it is a remarkable fact that inoculation with small-pox completely cured a protracted case of ophthalmia, as reported by Dezoteux;[38] and another case mentioned by Leroy,[39] which was also permanently cured.

A case of blindness, caused by suppression of tinea capitis, was entirely cured by small-pox, according to Klein.[40]

Small-pox was often known to produce deafness and asthma. But both of these tedious complaints were cured by it, when it had reached its height, as was observed by J. Fr. Closs.[41]

Swelling of the testicles, often of a serious kind, is a frequent effect of small-pox; and this disease, therefore, by means of its similitude, cured a large and hard swelling of the left testicle, caused by contusion; as was observed by Klein,[42] and a similar swelling of the testicles was seen by another observer[43] to be cured by it.

An affection of the bowels, resembling dysentery, is peculiar to the disturbances connected with small-pox; and, as observed by Fr. Went,[44] a case of dysentery was cured by variola, as a similar morbific potency.

It is well known that when variola is added to cow-pox, the former, by virtue of its superior intensity as well as its great similitude, will at once extinguish the latter homœopathically, and arrest its development. Cow-pox, on the other hand, having nearly attained its period of perfection, will, by its similitude, lessen to a great degree the virulence and danger of a subsequent eruption of small-pox, for which we have the testimony of Mühry,[45] and many others.

The lymph of inoculated cow-pox contains, besides its proper preventive vaccine matter, a principle capable of producing a general cutaneous eruption of different nature; this rarely consists of large pustules; but usually of small, dry, pointed pimples, seated upon red areolæ, intermingled with other circular, red blotches of skin, and is often accompanied by violent itching. In many children this eruption actually appears several days *before*, but more frequently *after*, the red areola of the cow-pox, and vanishes in a few days, leaving behind small, red, and hard spots of skin. By means of the similitude of this secondary miasm, the cow-pox cures similar, and often inveterate and troublesome cutaneous eruptions of children, after the vaccination has properly taken effect; and such homœopathic cures are perfect and durable, as many observers[46] testify.

Cow-pox known to produce the peculiar symptom of swelling of the arm,[47] cured, after its eruption, a *swollen* and half-paralyzed arm.[48]

The fever, accompanying cow-pox occurring about the time of the appearance of the red areola, homœopathically cured intermittent fever in two persons, as Hardege, Jr.,[49] reports; thereby confirming the observations of J. Hunter,[50] that two fevers (being similar) could not exist at one time in the body.*

Measles bear a strong resemblance to hooping-cough in regard to fever and the character of the cough, and hence Bosquillon[51] observed that, in an epidemic where both diseases prevailed, many children having already had the measles, escaped the hooping-cough in this epidemic. The measles would then and afterwards have protected all children against the contagion of hooping-cough, if this bore a more complete resemblance to measles; that is, if it were combined with a cutaneous eruption similar to that of measles. But,

---

* The examples of chronic diseases cured by means of the itch, which were mentioned in previous editions of the *Organon*, are only to be regarded as homœopathic cures in a limited sense, in consequence of the discoveries and disclosures contained in the first part of the book *On Chronic Diseases*. The severe and inveterate diseases (chronic dyspnœa, threatening suffocation, and cases of consumption), which were there seen to vanish, were originally of psoric origin. These dangerous symptoms proceeded from advanced psora, developed within the system. This was as usual again changed into the simple form of primitive itch-disease, by means of a recent infection of itch, by which the old diseases and their dangerous symptoms were removed. Hence, a transformation of this kind into the primitive form, deserves to be regarded as a homœopathic cure of advanced symptoms of inveterate psora, only because the new infection places the patient in a condition far more favorable for the speedy cure of the entire psora, by means of antipsoric remedies.

under these conditions, a certain number only could escape the hooping-cough in that epidemic, by the homœopathic agency of the measles. But when measles, characterized chiefly by the eruption, are brought in contact with a similar disease, they will undeniably extinguish and cure it homœopathically. In this manner an inveterate herpetic disease was at once cured[52] entirely and permanently (homœopathically) by the eruption of measles, as observed by Kortum.[53] A severe burning, rash-like eruption on the face, neck, and arms, of six years' standing, and renewed by every change of weather, was changed, by the accession of measles, into a swollen cutaneous surface; after the disappearance of the measles this skin disease was cured, and never returned.[54]

§ 47. The preceding examples contain the most distinct and convincing argument in regard to the kind of artificial, morbific potency (medicine) to be chosen by the physician, in order to accomplish rapid and permanent cures, according to the process observed in the course of nature.

§ 48. All of these examples prove that neither the efforts of nature, nor of the physician have ever been able to extinguish or cure a disease by means of a dissimilar morbific potency however powerful; but they prove that according to eternal and irrevocable laws of nature, which were hitherto misinterpreted, cures are made to result *alone from a morbific potency which is similar in symptoms, and somewhat superior in strength.*

§ 49. We would be able to discover a far greater number of instances of genuine, natural, homœopathic cures, if observers had devoted more attention to them, and also, if homœopathic auxiliary diseases (Hülfs-Krankheiten) were more frequent in nature.

§ 50. Great as the resources of nature are, she possesses no other homœopathic means of cure, besides a few miasmatic diseases of fixed character as auxiliaries (the itch), measles and small-pox.[55] Some of these in their capacity as curative agencies,[56] are more dangerous to life and more to be dreaded than the diseases which they cure; and others, like the itch, after having served their purpose of curing another disease, in turn require treatment to extinguish them. Both of these conditions render their application as homœopathic remedies difficult, uncertain, and dangerous; and besides, there are but few human diseases that would find their similar remedy in small-pox, measles, and itch. In the course of nature, therefore, only few evils are cured by means of these uncertain homœopathic agencies. The effects of such morbific potencies are fraught with danger and great suffering, because they cannot be diminished and controlled according to circumstances, like doses of medicine. But in order to rid a patient of a *similar* chronic evil, his body is completely invaded by an *entire*, dangerous, and tedious disease, such as small-pox, measles (and itch). Nevertheless we have seen that fortunate coincidences of this kind have resulted in excellent homœopathic cures, serving as so many irrefutable proofs of the existence of the great and only natural law: *to cure by means of similitude of symptoms.*

§ 51. Examples like the preceding were quite sufficient for the purpose of revealing this law of cure to the intelligent human mind. But man possesses great advantages over crude nature as observed in accidental phenomena; for he has at his disposal many thousands of homœopathic morbific potencies in the form of medicinal substances, in which nature abounds for the benefit of suffering fellow-beings. He discovers in them morbific agencies of every variety of effect, adapted to the countless, conceivable, and inconceivable natural diseases, for which they are capable of serving as homœopathic remedies. The power of these morbific potencies (medicinal substances), after successfully attaining their curative purpose, is overcome by the vital force, and vanishes of itself, without demanding another curative process for its subsequent expulsion, like psora. Artificial morbific potencies of that kind admit of being diluted, divided, and potentiated to the verge of infinity, and their dose may be diminished by the physician so as to retain only the necessary degree of superiority over the similar natural disease to be cured; therefore, the superiority of this method consists in the avoidance of every violent effect upon the organism, even in the treatment of inveterate chronic diseases; indeed, the result of this curative method becomes appreciable only in a gentle, imperceptible, but none the less rapid transition from the suffering of natural disease into the desired, enduring state of health.

§ 52. After becoming familiar with the above illustrative examples, no intelligent physician will continue to adhere to the usages of common, antiquated practice of attacking the body in its least diseased parts by (allopathic) medicines, such as purgatives, counter-stimulants, derivatives, etc.,[57] having no direct pathical (homœopathic) relation to the disease to be cured. Such a course produces a heterogeneous and dissimilar morbid condition, injurious to the patient; his strength is wasted by strong doses of compounds of mostly unknown drugs; and these are followed by no other result, than the one produced by the eternal laws of nature when, as in the cases quoted (or others of the same nature), two dissimilar diseases meet in the human organism; in which case *diseases are never cured, but always aggravated.* The effect of such treatment will be of three kinds: Example I (§ 36) proves that the older disease in possession of the body, repels the accessory, *dissimilar*, and weaker disease, according to the process of nature; in like manner, the natural disease remains unchanged under mild, though protracted allopathic treatment, which only debilitates the patient. Or, as illustrated by Example II (§ 38), the new and stronger disease only disguises and suspends for a short time the older, weaker, and *dissimilar* disease, according to the course pursued by nature; in the same manner, the violent action of strong allopathic medicines upon the body, will cause the earlier disease to yield apparently for a time; but only to return with equal intensity. Lastly, as illustrated by Example III (§ 40), in the course of nature, two dissimilar chronic diseases of equal intensity, may both become seated, and complicated within the organism. Hence, if a natural chronic disease is treated with dissimilar morbific potencies in the form of allopathic medicines, in large and frequently repeated doses, these, far from curing the original (dissimilar) chronic disease, will generate a new artificial disease by the side of the older one, and, as daily experience teaches, will only increase the illness of the patient, and render his case incurable.

§ 53. Genuine, gentle cures are accomplished, as we have seen, only by the principle of homœopathy. This principle, as we have already found (§§ 7–25) by conclusions derived from experience, truly furnishes the only method enabling human skill to cure diseases with great certainty, rapidity, and permanency; because this curative method rests upon an eternal, infallible law of nature.

§ 54. As above intimated (§§ 43–49), the course *pursued by homœopathy* must be the only correct one; because of the three ways in which it is possible to apply medicines in diseases, it is the only direct one leading to a gentle, certain, and permanent cure, without subsequent ill effects or debility. The true homœopathic method of cure is the only correct, the only direct, and the only possible means to be employed by human skill, as surely as it is possible to draw but one straight line between two given points.

§ 55. The next is the *allopathic or heteropathic* method of applying medicines in disease. This, though destitute of pathical relation to the actual disease within the body, is employed by its advocates to attack the soundest parts, in order, as they suppose, to remove the disease by derivation. This was hitherto the most common practice. I have discussed it in the Introduction,[58] and shall not touch upon it hereafter.

§ 56. Besides the two former, there is but one other way[59] of applying medicines in diseases; it is the *antipathic* (enantiopathic), or *palliative* method. This affords to the physician the opportunity of appearing as a benefactor, and the means of winning the confidence of the patient, by the delusion of temporary improvement. The following will illustrate the inefficacy and danger of this method as applied in diseases of a chronic nature. Although it is the only feature of the allopathic mode of treatment, bearing some visible relation to a portion of the symptoms of the natural disease, we find upon inquiry that the palliative method involves a misapplication (inversion) of principle to be most carefully avoided, that the patient may not be deceived.

§ 57. In order to apply the antipathic method, the common practitioner singles out the most troublesome symptom of a case, from among many others which he ignores altogether, and prescribes a remedy known to produce the exact counterpart of the symptoms to be cured, hoping thereby to cure the latter; and in this manner he may expect the most speedy palliative result. According to the rule *contraria contrariis*, dictated by the ancient school of medicine for more than fifteen hundred years, strong doses of opium are prescribed for all kinds of pain, because this remedy speedily benumbs sensation; and the very same remedy is given in diarrhœa, because it quickly checks the peristaltic motion of the intestines, and renders them insensible. The same remedy is also given in sleeplessness, because opium soon produces a soporific, heavy kind of sleep. Purgatives are prescribed in cases of habitual constipation and costiveness; and a burned hand is immersed in cold water, which by its coldness seems to remove the burning pain as if by magic. A patient suffering from chilliness, and deficiency of vital warmth, is placed in a warm bath, which temporarily warms his body. Those who suffer from chronic debility, are treated with wine, which produces only a brief period of temporary revival. Besides these, several other antagonistic (antipathic) measures are used, but their number is limited, because the common school of medicine is acquainted with the peculiar (primary) effect of a few remedies only.

§ 58. If, in judging this practice, I were to overlook its peculiar fault (see note to § 7) of providing *only in part for a single symptom*, that is, only for a small part of the whole disease, which would not be relieved by this method, nor the hopes of the patient realized, I would, nevertheless, consult experience to find a single instance of the employment of such antipathic remedies in obstinately chronic diseases, where the transient relief which they brought, was not followed by very perceptible aggravation, not only of a prominent symptom, but of the entire disease. After such inquiry, every attentive observer must admit that an aggravation will unexceptionally follow such temporary antipathic improvement; although the old school practitioner will interpret such an aggravation differently to the patient, perhaps by attributing it either to a new and violent change in the original disease, or to the appearance of a new one.[60]

§ 59. Such palliative antipathic remedies were never employed in allaying the prominent symptoms of protracted diseases, without being followed in a few hours by the contrary condition, *i. e.*, the return of the evil, often seriously aggravated. Coffee, producing exhilaration in its primary effect, was prescribed in cases of sleepiness, which would increase as soon as the effects of the coffee had subsided. Regardless of any other symptoms of the disease, nocturnal wakefulness was treated by opium, which, in its primary effect, produces heavy sleep; but in such cases the subsequent nights were attended with more sleeplessness than before. Also without reference to other signs of the disease, chronic diarrhœa was combated by opium, the primary effect of which is characterized by constipation; after checking the diarrhœa for a short time, it afterwards returns with greater severity. Violent and frequently returning pains of all kinds, are only suppressed for a short time by the benumbing effects of opium, after which they return increased beyond endurance; or some other far more serious evils are observed to take the place of those pains. The common practitioner knows of no better remedy for chronic night-cough than opium, which suppresses all kinds of irritation by its primary effect; it may, perhaps, silence the cough during the first night, only to be more aggravating in the following nights; and if it is again and again suppressed by highly increased doses of that palliative, fever and night-sweats will supervene. Weakness of the bladder, and consequent retention of urine, was hitherto treated with tincture of cantharides, an antipathic opposite, very irritating to the urinary passages; and, although it forced the evacuation of urine in the beginning, its subsequent effect was to diminish the irritability of the bladder to such a degree, as to make it powerless to contract, and finally to produce paralysis of that organ. It was hitherto customary to treat inveterate tendency to constipation, by stimulating the bowels to frequent evacuations with powerful purgatives and laxative salts; but their after-effects caused the constipation to become more obstinate. In ordinary practice it is usual to prescribe wine in chronic debility; but this merely excites in its primary effect, and consequently the strength declines to a lower degree in the after-effect. It is usual to see physicians endeavor to strengthen and warm a weakened and inactive stomach by bitter substances and heating spices; but while that organ is only excited by the primary effect of these palliatives, its inactivity becomes still more apparent in their after-effects. Warm baths are prescribed for chronic chilliness, and deficiency of vital warmth; but such patients are afterwards found to have become still weaker, colder, and more chilly. Severe burns are immediately relieved by application of cold water; but the burning pain is subsequently increased beyond endurance, and the inflammation extends and rises to a higher degree.[61] Chronic nasal catarrh is habitually treated by exciting the flow of mucus with errhines; but the fact is overlooked that the catarrh is constantly increased by this opposite (in its after-effect), and that the nose is still more obstructed. To limbs affected with chronic debility or partial paralysis, increased mobility is temporarily imparted by the application of potencies capable of exciting muscular action by their primary effect, such as electricity and galvanism; but the consequence (after-effect) proves to be total decline of muscular contractility, and complete paralysis. Bloodletting was commonly resorted to for the relief of chronic rush of blood to the head; but the result was always a greater degree of congestion. In the torpid state of bodily and mental organs, often found combined with stupor in many forms of typhus, the common school of medicine knew of no better remedy than valerian in large doses, because it is considered as one of the most powerful enlivening and exciting remedies; but that school was ignorant of the fact that this was only the primary effect, and that the after-effect (counter-effect), invariably reduced the organism to a greater degree of stupefaction and loss of mobility; leading eventually to fatal paralysis of bodily and mental organs. It escaped the attention of the old school that those cases in particular, which were most liberally fed with the antipathic valerian, usually terminated in death. The old-school physician rejoices[62] in his ability to retard for a few hours the small, rapid pulse in cachexias, by the primary effect of the first dose of purple foxglove; but soon its rapidity is renewed; repeated and increased doses lose their effect, and at length entirely cease to lessen the frequency of the pulse, which, on the contrary, now grows countless in the after-effect; sleep, appetite, and strength depart, and speedy dissolution is the *inevitable* consequence, unless insanity supervenes. Though unrecognized by false theories, deplorable results prove how frequently aggravations of diseases, and still more undesirable consequences, are produced by the after-effects of such opposite or antipathic remedies.

§ 60. In the presence of these evil results, necessarily proceeding from the antipathic use of medicines, the ordinary physician endeavors to escape the difficulty, as he thinks, by a stronger dose of the remedy, given during every new aggravation, which is succeeded by a lull of short duration. But as such transient relief makes a constant increase of the palliative dose necessary, this is followed by a new and more serious disorder, if not by danger to life, or by death itself. But the original disease, whether acute or chronic, *is never cured* by such means.

§ 61. *Had physicians correctly observed and considered the deplorable results of the antipathic application of medicines, they would long ago have discovered the great truth, that the true method of performing permanent cures must be the exact counterpart of such antipathic treatment.* They would have perceived that, whenever the opposite or antipathic administration of medicine produced a brief period of alleviation, this would subside, only to be followed by one of aggravation, and that, consequently, the process should have been reversed; that is to say, the *homœopathic application of medicines* according to their symptom-similitude, would have brought about a lasting and perfect cure, provided that, instead of large quantities of medicine, the most minute doses had been employed. Notwithstanding the experience of many centuries, physicians did not recognize this great and salutary truth. They appear to have ignored entirely the results of treatment above described, as well as the other fact, that no physician ever effected a permanent cure of an inveterate disease, unless some drug of *predominant* homœopathic effect had been by chance embodied in his prescription; nor were they able to comprehend that every rapid and perfect cure, accomplished by nature without the aid of human skill (§ 46), was always produced by a *similar* disease coming to the one already present.

§ 62. The following will explain the source of danger of antipathic treatment, as well as the efficacy of its counterpart, the homœopathic method. The examples chosen for this purpose, are derived from numerous observations which have entirely escaped notice before I called attention to them, although they were within the reach of every one, quite intelligible, and of vast importance in their relation to medical art.

§ 63. Every drug, like every other influence affecting vitality, alters the harmony of the vital force more or less, and produces a certain change in the state of health of the body for a longer or shorter space of time. This is called *primary effect.* Although a product of drug and vital force, it is probably due chiefly to the action of the drug. Our vital force, by means of its energy, endeavors to oppose this effect; the resulting conservative reaction is an automatic activity of the vital force, and is called *after-effect* or *counter-effect*.

§ 64. During the primary effect of artificial, morbific potencies (drugs) acting upon our healthy body, our vital force seems to be only receptive or passive, and appears to be compelled, as it were, to receive the impressions made upon it by the drug, and to allow the state of health to be altered by it. Thereupon the vital force seems to rally, and the result may be twofold: first, if the possibility exists of producing the exact counterpart of the primary effect, the vital force calls it forth in form of the exact opposite state of feeling (counter-effect), which is quite in proportion to the energy of the vital force, and to the intensity of the primary impression made upon it by the artificial morbific potency or medicine; or, secondly, where nature affords no exact opposite condition to the primary effect, the vital force apparently endeavors to become neutralized (sich zu indifferenziren), *i. e.*, to put forth its superior strength in extinguishing the impression made upon it by the drug, thereby reëstablishing the normal state of health, which is the *after-effect*, or *curative effect*.

§ 65. Examples of the *first* instance referred to, are familiar to everybody. A hand bathed in hot water is at first much warmer than the other unbathed hand (primary effect); but removed from the hot water, and having been well dried, it will after awhile grow cold, and at last much colder than the other hand (after-effect). A person heated by violent bodily exercise (primary effect) will afterwards feel chills and rigors (after-effect). To a person heated by drinking too much wine (primary effect), every breath of air will seem too cold next day (counter-effect of the organism, after-effect). An arm immersed for a length of time in very cold water, is at first much paler and colder (primary effect) than the other, but withdrawn from the water and dried, it will become not only warmer than the other, but even hot, red, and inflamed (after-effect, counter-effect of the vital force). The primary effect of strong coffee is excessive wakefulness, but lassitude and sleepiness will remain long afterwards (counter-effect, after-effect), if this wakefulness is temporarily removed by the repeated use of coffee (palliative). The heavy, soporific sleep produced by opium (primary effect), will be followed next night by greater sleeplessness (counter-effect, after-effect). After constipation produced by opium (primary effect) follows diarrhœa (after-effect), and after purging (primary effect) excited by drugs which stimulate the bowels, constipation and costiveness (after-effect) may be observed for several days. And thus, whenever the possibility actually exists, the exact counterpart is always produced by our vital force in its after-effect, following each primary effect of a large dose of any potency, by which the feelings of the healthy body are seriously deranged.

§ 66. A conspicuous opposite or after-effect is imperceptible during the action of very minute, homœopathic doses of alterative potencies (drugs, medicines) in the healthy body. Although minute doses, when closely observed, may be seen to produce a perceptible primary effect, the living organism sets up only so much counter-effect (after-effect) as is required for the re-establishment of the normal condition.

§ 67. Incontrovertible truths like the preceding, spontaneously offered by nature and experience, explain to us the salutary process of homœopathic cures, and expose, at the same time, the objections to palliative treatment of the sick, by means of the antipathic effects of medicines.[63]

§ 68. We learn from homœopathic cures that, after the extinction of the natural disease, there is apt to linger in the system a remnant of the drug disease engendered by the minute doses of medicine (§§ 275–287) required by this method of cure, and which were just sufficient to overcome and to supersede the similar, natural disease by the similitude of their symptoms. But we also learn that this remnant of drug disease is very transient, and vanishes easily and quickly on account of the extreme minuteness of the dose; this prevents the vital force from being aroused to a greater degree of counteraction against this slight artificial effect than is requisite for the restoration of feelings to the standard of health. That is, for the purpose of *complete* recovery, the vital force needs to make but a slight additional exertion to overcome the effects of the medicine, after the extinction of the disease for which it was given. (This may serve to explain the *second* instance in § 65.)

§ 69. Precisely the reverse of this, takes place in antipathic (palliative) treatment. The drug symptom opposed by the physician to a symptom of the disease (*e. g.*, insensibility and stupor, the primary effect of opium in opposition to acute pain), is not allopathic in relation to the latter. There evidently exists a relation between drug-symptom and disease-symptom, but it is *reversed.* The extinction of the disease-symptom is, in this case, to be accomplished by an opposite drug-symptom, which is quite impossible. It is true that the antipathic medicine acts upon the same diseased region of the body, and with the same degree of certainty as the homœopathic medicine selected on account of its similar morbific effect, but the former being an opposite to the symptom of the disease, it only obscures the latter, and renders it imperceptible for a short time. The vital force perceives no disagreeable sensation (neither from the symptoms of the disease, nor from that of the opponent drug) during the first moment of the effect produced by the opponent palliative, because both appear to have cancelled, or to have dynamically neutralized each other; as, *e. g.*, the benumbing power of opium seems to neutralize pain. During the first minutes of palliative effect, the vital force feels as if in health, perceiving neither the benumbing effect of opium, nor the pain of the disease. But since the opposite drug effect is not a most similar (stronger, artificial) disease, influencing the vital force like the effect of a remedy chosen according to the homœopathic method, it cannot occupy the place of the natural, morbid disturbance in the organism; and consequently the effect of the palliative medicine, differing totally in contrast with the natural disease, will be unable to extinguish the latter. Although, by means of the apparent dynamic neutralization[64] of the palliative, the vital force seems at first to be made insensible to the morbid disturbance, the effect of the palliative will, nevertheless, subside of its own accord, like every drug effect. But it will leave the disease to remain as it was; for, in order to produce the semblance of relief, it had to be administered in large doses like all palliatives, and as such it incites the vital force to a state of opposition to this palliative medicine (§§ 63–65). This opposition, though the counterpart of the palliative, resembles the natural disease still present and uncured, but necessarily intensified and increased[65] by the additional activity which the vital force was obliged to maintain in counteracting the palliative. Therefore, after the decline of the palliative drug effect, the obnoxious symptoms (a mere part of the disease) will be found to have been aggravated *in proportion to the size of the palliative dose.* And, to continue the same example, the larger the dose of opium is, for the purpose of obscuring the pain, so much the more will the latter be increased beyond its original intensity as soon as the opium has ceased to act.[66]

§ 70. After these premises, the following points must be admitted as true:

1st. All that a physician may regard as curable in diseases, consists entirely in the complaints of the patient, and the morbid changes of his health perceptible to the senses; that is to say, it consists entirely in the totality of symptoms through which the disease expresses its demand for the appropriate remedy; while, on the other hand, every fictitious or obscure, internal cause and condition, or imaginary, material, morbific matter are not objects of treatment.

2d. This change of health (discord of feeling) which we call disease, can only be changed back (umstimmen) to the normal state by means of medicines, the curative power of which, consequently, consists in their ability to alter the state of feelings; *i. e.*, in the production of peculiar, morbid symptoms, recognized most distinctly and purely by testing these medicines upon the bodies of healthy persons.

3d. According to experience, natural disease cannot be cured by medicines producing by themselves, in healthy persons, a morbid condition *dissimilar* to and different from that of the disease to be cured. It is, therefore, incurable by allopathic treatment, and even nature herself never cures natural disease by superadding another disease, dissimilar to, though of much greater intensity than the first.

4th. Experience also teaches that only transient relief is procured by medicines inclined to generate in a healthy person, an artificial symptom which is the exact opposite of certain symptoms, peculiar to the natural disease to be cured. And we also learn that such medicines can never cure an inveterate disease, without always creating a subsequent aggravation of the same. On this account this antipathic, palliative process is entirely inappropriate in its application to chronic and serious diseases.

5th. The only really salutary treatment is that of the *homœopathic* method, according to which the totality of symptoms of a natural disease is combated by a medicine in commensurate dose, capable of creating in the healthy body, symptoms most similar to those of the natural disease. And as diseases are only dynamic disturbances of the vital force, they are overcome without additional suffering, and having been perfectly and permanently extinguished, they must cease to exist. Nature when left to her own resources, furnishes examples in the form of accidental cures; as, for instance, when a new and similar disease is added to the older one, this is permanently extinguished and cured.

§ 71. Now, since it is subject to no further doubt, that human diseases consist merely in groups of certain symptoms, and that these may be extinguished, and the system restored to health only by means of a medicinal substance possessing the power of producing artificial, morbid symptoms, similar to the disease (whereon rests the process of every genuine cure), the business of curing will depend on the solution of the following problems:

I. How does the physician gain the knowledge of disease, necessary for the purpose of cure?

II. How does he gain his knowledge of the morbific power of drugs, as the implements designed for the cure of natural diseases?

III. How does he apply these artificial, morbific potencies (drugs) most effectively in the cure of diseases?

§ 72. Regarding the first point, the following may serve as a general illustration. Diseases peculiar to mankind, are of two classes. The first includes rapid, morbid processes caused by abnormal states and derangements of the vital force; such affections usually run their course within a brief period of variable duration, and are called *acute* diseases. The second class embraces diseases which often seem trifling and imperceptible in the beginning; but which, in a manner peculiar to themselves, act deleteriously upon the living organism, dynamically deranging the latter, and insidiously undermining its health to such a degree, that the automatic energy of the vital force, designed for the preservation of life, can only make imperfect and ineffectual resistance to these diseases in their beginning, as well as during their progress. Unable to extinguish them without assistance, the vital force is powerless to prevent their growth or its own gradual deterioration, resulting in the final destruction of the organism. These are called *chronic* diseases, and are originated by infection with a chronic miasm.

§ 73. Acute diseases likewise admit of division into

several classes. The first are those which attack single individuals; they are occasioned by hurtful influences to which the patient happened to be exposed. Excesses in sensual enjoyment, or deprivation of the same; violent physical impressions; exposure to cold; overheating; excessive muscular exertion; physical or mental excitement, etc., give rise to acute febrile diseases. They are, however, in reality but transient aggravations of latent psora, which returns to its dormant condition of its own accord, provided the acute disease was not too violent and speedily relieved. The second class includes sporadic diseases which attack several persons simultaneously in isolated localities. They are engendered by meteoric or telluric agencies, to the morbific influence of which, only few persons are susceptible at a time. Next to this class come the *epidemic* diseases, which attack many persons at the same time; they arise from the same cause, and individual cases resemble each other; these diseases usually become infectious (*contagious*) when they pervade crowded districts, where they create fevers[67] of a distinct kind; and as the cases of disease are of like origin, they are also alike in their manifestations; but if left to themselves, they will, within a limited period, terminate in recovery or death, as the case may be. War, inundations, and famine frequently give rise and growth to such diseases. They often appear in the form of distinct *acute miasms*, that invariably appear in the same form (whence they are known by a traditional name). Some of them attack the same person but once in life, like small-pox, measles, hooping-cough, the once well-known smooth, light-red scarlet fever[68] of Sydenham, the mumps, etc., or they may repeatedly attack the same person; like the levantine plague, returning in nearly the same form; the yellow fever infecting districts on the seacoast; the Asiatic cholera, etc.

§ 74. It is a matter of regret that we are still obliged to count among chronic diseases very common affections which are to be regarded as the result of allopathic treatment, and the continual use of violent, heroic medicines, in large and increasing doses. Examples of that kind are: the abuse of calomel, corrosive sublimate, mercurial ointment, nitrate of silver, iodine and its ointments, opium, valerian, Peruvian bark and quinia, digitalis, prussic acid, sulphur and sulphuric acid, the use of purgatives persisted in for years, bloodletting, leeches, issues, setons, etc. Such wanton treatment weakens the organism; or, if not entirely prostrated, it is gradually and abnormally deranged, according to the individual character of each drug. During this exhausting and deleterious treatment, the vital force is compelled, in defence of life, to alter the entire organism. Accordingly, it diminishes or increases the irritability, or sensibility of various parts; it produces hypertrophy or atrophy; softening or induration in certain organs, resulting eventually in destruction, or, at least, in organic lesions (deformities) of external or internal parts.[69] These are some of the results of the efforts of nature to protect the organism against complete destruction, to which it is exposed by the constant renewal of aggressive treatment with pernicious substances.

§ 75. Instances of ruined health, resulting from allopathic treatment, are very common in modern times. They constitute the most pitiable, and incurable of chronic diseases, and it is to be feared that remedies will probably never be found, or invented for the cure of such conditions, when they have reached a certain degree of severity.

§ 76. It is only through homœopathy that Providence has vouchsafed to us the means of curing natural diseases; but not those chronic external and internal lesions and deformities, wantonly forced upon the human organism by unskilful treatment, and pernicious medicines. Nevertheless, if proper measures are directed against the chronic miasm, perhaps lurking in the system, the vital force might still be made to undo much of the mischief, provided it had not been weakened by treatment to such an extent as to prevent it from being undisturbed for a sufficient number of years, required for the accomplishment of the enormous task. The art of healing is not, and never will be perfected so far, as to enable us to rectify the countless ill effects so often observable after allopathic treatment of the sick.

§ 77. The name of chronic diseases does not apply to those which are produced by constant exposure to *avoidable* noxious influences; by indulgence in habitual excesses in eating, drinking, and various kinds of health-destroying debauchery; nor to those diseases which result from constant want of the necessaries of life; unhealthy dwellings, particularly in marshy localities; diseases peculiar to the inhabitants of cellars or other confined places, suffering from want of fresh air and exercise; nor those which are the result of overtaxed body and mind, or continued mortifications and trouble, etc. Provided there is no other chronic miasm pervading the organism, unhealthy conditions like the above, will vanish of their own accord, under an improved mode of living, and they do not deserve the name of chronic diseases.

§ 78. True, natural, *chronic* diseases are those which owe their origin to a chronic miasm; they constantly extend, and, notwithstanding the most carefully regulated mental and bodily habits, they will never cease to torment their victim with constantly renewed suffering to the end of his life, if left to themselves without the aid of specific remedies for their relief. These are the most numerous, and the source of great suffering to the human race; the most robust constitution, the best of habits, and the greatest energy of unaided vital force are unable to resist them.

§ 79. Hitherto only syphilis was known to some extent as one of these chronic miasmatic diseases, which, if left uncured, will become extinct only with life itself. Sycosis (cauliflower-excrescences) if left to itself uncured, is likewise inextinguishable by the vital force, and was not hitherto recognized as an internal, chronic, miasmatic disease of peculiar nature, as it undoubtedly is. Without noticing the perpetual evils entailed by it, the destruction of the cutaneous excrescences alone, was considered as a cure of the entire disease.

§ 80. But psora, as a chronic miasm, is of incomparably greater significance than either of the above-named chronic miasms. While venereal chancre and the cauliflower excrescences mark the internal, specific nature of the two former diseases, psora, after complete infection of the entire organism, indicates its origin from an internal and monstrous chronic miasm, by a peculiar cutaneous eruption, sometimes consisting merely in a few pimples combined with intolerable tickling, voluptuous itching, and specific odor. Psora is the only real, *fundamental cause* and source of all the other countless forms of disease,[70] figuring as peculiar and definite diseases in books on pathology, under the names of nervous debility, hysteria, hypochondriasis, mania, melancholy, idiocy, madness, epilepsy and convulsions of all kinds, softening of the bones (*rachitis*), scoliosis and kyphosis, caries of the bones, cancer, varices, pseudoplasms, gout, hæmorrhoids, icterus and cyanosis, dropsy, amenorrhœa, hæmorrhages from the stomach, nose, lungs, bladder, or uterus; asthma and suppuration of the lungs; impotence and sterility; sick headache (hemicrania); deafness; cataract and glaucoma; renal calculus; paralysis; deficiency of the special senses, and pains of every variety.

§ 81. Without doubt this ancient, smouldering contagion has gradually passed through several hundreds of generations, and many millions of human organisms, thus reaching an incredible degree of development. We may, therefore, comprehend in a measure, how it became developed into countless forms of disease peculiar to the great human race; particularly when we contemplate the mass of circumstances[71] which produce and favor the formation of so great a variety of chronic diseases (secondary symptoms of psora). Considering the endless diversity in human beings, differing among each other in regard to bodily constitutions of countless variety, it is not a matter of surprise that ordinary and manifold, noxious influences, acting from within and from without upon so great a variety of individuals pervaded by psoric miasm, should also produce various disorders, lesions, and disturbances of health, which have hitherto been known by a long list of *names* in the old works on pathology,[72] where they figure as distinct diseases.

§ 82. Although the discovery of the great source of chronic diseases, as well as the introduction of more specific homœopathic remedies, for psora in particular, has advanced the healing art several steps in its ability to cure most chronic diseases; nevertheless the indispensable obligation of the homœopathic physician to carefully comprehend every discernible symptom and peculiarity of the case, for the purpose of forming an indication for each chronic disease, remains in force as it was before the discovery of psora. Genuine cures of these, or any other diseases, are not to be accomplished without rigid, special treatment (individualization) of each case; but in pursuing the investigation, it is necessary to distinguish whether the disease is of *acute*, or of *chronic* origin. In the first instance the principal symptoms are more quickly perceived and recognized; the whole presents itself spontaneously to the senses; and much less time is consumed by inquiry,[73] and in noting the characteristic features (image) of the case, than in the laborious examination of the symptoms of chronic diseases that have gradually progressed for several years.

§ 83. Individualization in the *investigation of a case of disease*, demands, on the part of the physician, principally unbiassed judgment and sound senses, attentive observation, and fidelity in noting down the image of the disease. For this purpose, I will give the following general directions, which may serve the examining physician as guides in each given case.

§ 84. The patient narrates the history of his complaints; his attendants communicate what they have heard him complain of, and describe his behavior, and other circumstances they have observed. The physician observes by means of sight, hearing, and touch, what is changed and abnormal about the patient, and writes down everything in precisely the same expressions used by the patient and his attendants. He quietly allows them to finish their story, if possible without interruption, unless they digress upon irrelevant topics,[74] only requesting them at the outset to speak slowly, to allow him to takes notes of the speaker's words.

§ 85. At the end of each statement of the patient or attendants, the physician should begin a new sentence in writing, so that the symptoms may be noted separately, one beneath the other. This will permit of subsequent additions to statements which were indefinite at first, but afterwards repeated more distinctly.

§ 86. When the patient and attendants have ended their statements of their own accord, the physician supplies each symptom with a more precise definition, to be obtained by reading over the single symptoms communicated to him, and here and there instituting particular inquiry; for instance: at what time did this attack occur? Was it some time before the present medicine? Was it during its use? Or was it some days after discontinuing the medicine? Describe exactly what kind of pain or sensation occurred, and where was the exact place? Did the pain come in single paroxysms, at different times? Or was it lasting and uninterrupted? How long did it last? At what time of the day or night, and in what position of the body was the pain most violent; or altogether absent? In this manner every attack or circumstance alluded to by the patient, should be made the subject of careful inquiry and description.

§ 87. In this manner the physician obtains a closer definition of each statement, without predetermining[75] the patient's reply, and avoids his answer by simple "yes" or "no." Otherwise the patient might be induced to affirm or deny facts, to state only partial truths, or to represent his case in a different light for the sake of convenience; or to please the physician, and thus to produce a false impression regarding the symptoms of his disease which, again, would lead to an improper mode of treatment.

§ 88. If, in these voluntary statements, the patient neglects to mention the condition of certain parts and functions of his body, or of his state of mind, the physician should endeavor to refresh the patient's memory concerning his observations on these subjects.[76] But the inquiry should be pursued without leading questions, so that the patient or attendant may be obliged to make special statements.

§ 89. After the patient (who should be trusted with regard to the expression of his feelings, except in imaginary diseases) has properly completed the picture of his disease, and given the desired information by voluntary and unbiassed statements, the physician (if he considers the information still imperfect) may find it necessary to ask some specific questions.[77]

§ 90. After having taken notes of the patient's statements, the physician should proceed to make a memorandum of what he has himself observed upon the patient,[78] and inquire as to the peculiarities of the patient in times of health.

§ 91. Symptoms and sensations experienced by the patient during some previous use of medicines, do not furnish a true image of the disease; those symptoms and complaints, however, suffered by the patient *before the use of medicines, for several days, or after their omission,* truthfully portray the original form of the disease, and should be particularly noted by the physician. When the disease is an inveterate one, or if the patient has persisted in the use of medicine up to this time, he may omit the same entirely, or something of an unmedicinal kind may be given him, while the rigorous examination of the case is postponed until the unadulterated, permanent symptoms of the chronic disorder can be ascertained in their purity, and a true picture of the disease obtained.

§ 92. But, if the disease is very acute, the urgent nature of which suffers no delay, and if the physician finds no time to seek information concerning the symptoms observed before medicines had been resorted to, he may have to accept the morbid state as modified by drugs, and to embrace it in one record. A disease, complicated by the effects of drugs improperly employed, is usually more serious and dangerous than the original evil, and, therefore, urgently demands appropriate measures for its relief; these are found in carefully selected homœopathic remedies, which are able to overcome the complicated disease, and perhaps to avert the danger caused by the drugs.

§ 93. If the acute or chronic disease is the result of some unfortunate incident which the patient hesitates to disclose, either spontaneously or upon careful inquiry, his friends, if privately appealed to, will usually furnish the desired information.[79]

§ 94. The investigation of the condition of chronic diseases should be conducted with particular reference to the circumstances of the patient; his usual occupation, habits of living, his diet, his domestic relations, etc., should be carefully considered, in order to discover to what extent errors of living participated in the production and maintenance of the disease, and what will be the appropriate means of their ultimate removal, and of the restoration of health.[80]

§ 95. In chronic diseases, the investigation of the above-named, and all other symptoms, should be conducted as carefully and circumstantially as possible, and made to penetrate the minutest details, because they are most peculiar and most unlike those of acute affections, and also because they can never be too accurately considered for the purpose of successful treatment. Again, chronic patients are so inured to suffering, that circumstances, however characteristic and decisive in the selection of the remedy, are rarely, if at all, mentioned by them, but rather considered as a part of their unavoidable condition. Such patients forget that these are deviations from health, the true consciousness of which, they have nearly lost during fifteen or twenty years of suffering; and it rarely occurs to them, that these secondary symptoms, and other small or great deviations from the healthy condition, might be connected with the main disease.

§ 96. It is worthy of remark that the temperament of patients is often abnormally affected; so that some, particularly hypochondriacs, and other sensitive and intolerant persons, are apt to represent their complaints in too strong a light, and to define them by exaggerated expressions,[81] hoping thereby to induce the physician to redouble his efforts.

§ 97. But there are persons of another kind of temperament, who withhold many complaints from the physician, partly from false modesty, timidity or bashfulness; and who state their case in obscure terms; or who consider many of their symptoms as too insignificant to mention.

§ 98. Although it is very desirable to obtain the patient's own statement regarding his complaints and sensations, and to observe particularly the expressions he uses in describing his sufferings, the history of which is apt to be more or less misrepresented by friends and attendants, it is equally true that the investigation of all diseases, especially of the chronic, demands great caution, reflection, knowledge of human nature, careful inquiry, and unlimited patience, in order to obtain a true and complete record of these diseases with all their details.

§ 99. On the whole, the physician experiences far less difficulty in the examination of acute diseases, or those of recent origin, because every new and striking incident and deviation from recent health, is still fresh in the memory of the patient and his attendants. Although the physician should be well acquainted with a case like this, it requires a less urgent inquiry, since the most important facts are readily communicated to him.

§ 100. In the exploration of the totality of symptoms of epidemic and sporadic diseases, it is a matter of no importance whether or not anything of a similar kind, or name, ever occurred before. Neither the novelty, nor peculiarity of such an epidemic makes any difference in the manner of its examination or cure, because, under all circumstances, the physician should presuppose the true image of any prevalent disease to be new and unknown; he should, therefore, investigate it anew and thoroughly by itself, if he claims to be a master of the art of healing, who neither allows conjectures to stand in the place of actual perceptions, nor ever presumes to know the particulars of a case of disease intrusted to him, without previous careful inquiry concerning all of its manifestations. This is particularly applicable to every prevailing epidemic, which is in many respects a phenomenon of peculiar kind, that will be found, on careful examination, to differ much from all previous epidemics to which specific names are erroneously applied; excepting, however, the epidemics engendered by an unvarying contagion, such as small-pox, measles, etc.

§ 101. It is possible that a physician meeting with the first case of a certain epidemic, should fail to perceive at once its perfect image, because every collective disease of this kind will not manifest the totality of its symptoms and character, until several cases have been carefully observed. But after having observed one or two cases of this kind, a physician accustomed to exact observation, may approach the true condition of the epidemic so closely, that he is enabled to construe a characteristic image of the same, and even to discover the appropriate homœopathic remedy.

§ 102. By writing down the symptoms of several cases of this kind, the sketch of the disease will gradually become more complete; without being enlarged by additional phrases, it will be more closely defined (more characteristic), and made to embrace more of the peculiarity of this collective disease. General signs, such as want of appetite, sleeplessness, etc., are specified and defined, while the more prominent and special symptoms which are rare in this, and peculiar only to a few diseases, will be made conspicuous by proper notation, and will constitute the characteristics of the epidemic.[82] The individuals who suffer from a prevalent epidemic, are apt to be affected *alike,* because each case arises from the same source; nevertheless, neither the totality and scope of such an epidemic, nor the totality of its symptoms (the knowledge of which is necessary for the purpose of obtaining a perfect image of the disease, and of selecting the suitable homœopathic remedy for the same) are to be observed upon a single patient; such knowledge is only to be obtained, in a perfect manner, by observation of the affections of several patients of different bodily constitutions.

§ 103. The method of investigating acute, epidemic diseases, was also employed by me in the examination of the unvarying, miasmatic, chronic diseases, particularly in the study of psora. These diseases required much greater care and diligence than had hitherto been devoted to them, in order to discover the whole range of their symptoms. In these cases, also, one patient presents only a portion of those symptoms, while a second and a third, etc., exhibits still another set, which constitutes, as it were, but a detached fragment of the totality of symptoms belonging to the entire chronic disease. A complex like this, particularly that of psora, could only be ascertained by examining *a great many* chronic cases. Without a complete image construed out of the totality of these symptoms, it would be impossible to discover the medicines (particularly the antipsorics) for the homœopathic cure of the entire disease; but having done so, these medicines prove to be the true remedies for individual cases of chronic evils of this kind.

§ 104. When all of the prominent and characteristic symptoms, collectively forming an image of a case of chronic, or of any other disease, have been carefully committed to writing,[83] the most difficult part of the labor will have been accomplished. The image which has now been construed, forms the basis of treatment, particularly of chronic diseases. This image is always accessible to the physician, whom it enables to oversee all its parts, to mark its characteristic signs representing the disease, and to prescribe a homœopathic remedy; that is, one which in its effects on healthy persons, produces symptoms strikingly similar to those of the disease. This remedy is found by comparing the lists of symptoms of all remedies that have become known in regard to their purely pathogenetic effects. Upon subsequent inquiry concerning the effects of the remedy, and the changes of feelings it has produced in the patient, and after having made a new record of the case, the physician will only have to omit from his diary that portion of the original group of symptoms which has been improved, and to note what remains, or what has subsequently appeared in the form of new symptoms.

§ 105. *The second point* pertaining to the duties of the true physician relates to the *discovery of the material necessary for the cure of natural diseases;* that is, to the investigation of the morbific power of drugs. Having attained this object, it will then be possible to select a medicine from the list of whose symptoms an artificial disease can be construed, which should be as similar as possible to the principal symptoms of the natural disease to be cured.

§ 106. The entire range of disease-producing power of each drug, must be known; that is, all morbid symptoms and changes of the state of health which each drug is capable of producing by itself in healthy persons, should have been observed in its fullest extent, before we may hope to find and to select, from among the medicines thus investigated, the truly homœopathic remedies for most natural diseases.

§ 107. If, for the purpose of investigation, drugs are given only to *sick persons,* and even if these drugs are administered singly and in simple forms, little or nothing of a definite kind will be seen of their pure effects, because the changes of health which these drugs may actually be expected to produce, would be mingled with the symptoms of the natural disease, so as to become obscured, and rarely to be distinctly visible.

§ 108. Hence, there is no other way of obtaining reliable knowledge of the peculiar power by virtue of which, drugs affect and alter human health; *i. e.*, there is no other safe, or more natural method of accomplishing this object, than to administer each drug separately, and in moderate quantity, *to healthy persons,* by way of experiment, in order to discover what changes, symptoms, and signs of its effect, that is, what elements of disease each is able to produce, and inclined to excite[84] by itself in the condition of the body and mind. For it has been shown (§§ 24–27) that the curative power of medicines depends alone upon their power of altering the state of health of the human organism, and that this power is revealed only in the observations made upon the latter.

§ 109. I was the first to pursue this course with perseverance, prompted and supported by perfect conviction of the great and beneficent truth, that human diseases can only be cured with certainty[85] by means of the homœopathic administration of medicines.[86]

§ 110. Next to this, I observed that the morbific, or toxical properties hitherto mentioned by authors as the effects of medicinal substances, which happened by mistake, or for suicidal or criminal purposes, to have been consumed in large quantities by healthy persons, coincided well with my own observations while experimenting with the same substances upon myself and other healthy persons. Authors generally report these cases of poisoning as proofs of the injurious effects of these powerful substances, and as a warning against them. When the patient happened to recover from the effects of drugs under the use of antidotes, some quote these cases as proofs of skill, while others report the fatal effects of those substances, by way of explaining their want of success; in this case, those substances are designated as poisons. None of these observers suspected that the symptoms reported only as proofs of the injurious and poisonous qualities of drugs, distinctly pointed to their medicinal power of extinguishing similar symptoms arising from natural diseases. None ever perceived that the disease-producing power of drugs could be made available homœopathically in the cure of diseases. None ever discovered that the only possible way of exploring the medicinal virtues of drugs is based exclusively upon the observation of the changes produced by them in the healthy body; because the actual and peculiar curative powers of drugs can never be recognized *a priori* through the sophistry of wiseacres, nor through odor, taste, and appearance of medicines; neither through chemical tests, nor through the use of several drugs, combined in one mixture (recipe), administered in disease. It was never suspected that such reports of drug-diseases would in future form the first rudiments of a true and pure science of *Materia Medica*, which had hitherto consisted merely of false suppositions and fiction, and which, therefore, had never existed in reality.[87]

§ 111. The agreement of my own observations of pure drug-effects (although made without regard to therapeutics), with those of older authors, as well as the agreement of the observations of various other writers among themselves, will easily convince us that medicinal substances, in producing morbid changes of the healthy human body, *act in obedience to fixed and eternal laws of nature*, by virtue of which laws, they are enabled to generate *certain definite morbid symptoms;* and that each drug produces particular symptoms, according to its peculiarity.

§ 112. In older descriptions of the fatal effects of overdoses of medicines, it is often to be noticed that the close of such deplorable accidents was marked by certain effects, which were of very different nature from those witnessed at the beginning of the case. These symptoms which are called forth in opposition to the *primary effect* (§ 63), or actual operation of drugs upon the vital force of the organism, are its counter-effect, or *after-effect* (§§ 62–67). But these are rarely if ever perceived after moderate doses administered to healthy persons for the purpose of experiment; and they are altogether absent after minute doses. During the homœopathic, curative process, the living organism exhibits only that degree of counteraction against these minute doses, which is required to reëstablish the natural state of health (§ 67).

§ 113. Only narcotic drugs should be regarded as exceptions to this rule. As these destroy sensibility and sensation, as well as irritability, in their primary effect, a heightened state both of sensibility and of irritability is frequently observed in healthy persons, as an *after-effect* following the administration of narcotics, even in moderate doses.

§ 114. With these exceptions, therefore, experiments made with moderate doses of other drugs upon healthy persons, exhibit only primary effects; *i. e.*, those symptoms by means of which a drug affects or deranges the healthy state, and produces in the organism a morbid condition of variable duration.

§ 115. Some drugs are known to produce certain effects which, in regard to certain minor features, appear to be the counterparts of other symptoms that may have appeared before, as well as after, the former. But notwithstanding this difference, these contrary symptoms are not to be regarded as actual *after-affects* or counter-effects of the vital force; because they merely indicate an alternation or fluctuation (Wechselzustand) of the various stages of the primary effect; on which account they are called alternating effects (Wechselwirkungen).

§ 116. Some symptoms are frequently produced by drugs in many healthy persons who try them; others are produced in but a few; others, again, are extremely rare.

§ 117. The so-called idiosyncrasies may be said to belong to the latter class. This term is applied to peculiar constitutions which, though otherwise healthy, are inclined to be more or less morbidly affected by certain things which *appear* to make no impression, and to produce no change in many other individuals.[88] But this want of susceptibility *is only apparent, not real.* In this, as well as in the production of all other morbific effects, two conditions necessarily exist: first, there is the active power residing in the drug; and secondly, the vital force of the organism possesses the faculty of being affected by the active principle of the drug. Consequently, the remarkable diseases arising from so-called idiosyncrasies, cannot be attributed alone to this particular kind of bodily constitution; but they should be considered as due also to the effect of drugs which possess the power of influencing every living organism; but with the exception, that some healthy constitutions are inclined to be more seriously and perceptibly affected than others. The fact that drugs prove to be homœopathic, curative remedies[89] in all cases of disease (although only seemingly in all idiosyncrasies), presenting symptoms similar to those which the drugs are capable of producing, tends to prove that they actually have the power of affecting all persons.

§ 118. Each drug manifests particular effects in the human body; and no other drug will produce effects of exactly the same kind.[90]

§ 119. There is no doubt that every species of plant differs from other species and genus in exterior form, in the peculiar manner of life and growth, in taste and odor; nor is there any doubt that every mineral, and every salt differs in its external and internal, chemical and physical properties, which alone should have prevented one from being mistaken for the other. It is, therefore, equally certain that all of them differ, and deviate among each other in their morbific as well as in their healing properties;[91] and that each of these substances acts in a manner so peculiar and distinct, and produces alternations in the state of health and feelings of man, so different from all others, as to prevent them from being confounded.[92]

§ 120. Medicines should, therefore, be distinguished from each other with scrupulous accuracy, and proved by pure and careful experiments with regard to their powers, and true effects upon the healthy body. For, upon the accuracy of this test (proving), depend life and death, sickness and health of human beings. The test should be so conducted as to result in the acquisition of accurate knowledge of drugs, as well as to avoid every mistake in using them in diseases; for, the unerring selection of remedies is the only condition for the speedy and permanent return of health of body and soul, the highest gift bestowed on man.

§ 121. In proving drugs in regard to their effects upon the healthy body, it should be remembered that the strong, so-called heroic substances, even in small doses, have the property of effecting changes in the health, even of robust persons. Those of milder power should be given in considerable doses in these experiments; and those of least activity, in order to cause their effect to become perceptible, should be tried only upon healthy, but sensitive and susceptible persons.

§ 122. As the success of the art of healing, and the welfare of all coming generations, depend entirely on these experiments, only such drugs should be employed which are perfectly reliable in regard to the purity, genuineness, and full strength.

§ 123. Each of these drugs must be taken into the system in a perfectly simple, and unartificial form. The juice pressed out of indigenous plants, should be mixed with a little alcohol, to prevent its deterioration; but foreign herbs should be used in the form of powder, or freshly prepared alcoholic tincture, mixed with several parts of water. Salts and gums, however, should be dissolved in water before administration. If a plant is to be obtained only in the dried state, and if its powers are naturally weak, the experiment may be made with the infusion, prepared by pouring boiling water over the herb previously powdered, whereby its virtues are extracted. Such infusions should be drank immediately after their preparation while warm, because all expressed juices, and watery infusions of plants, will rapidly pass into fermentation and deterioration without the addition of spirits, and will then lose their medicinal properties.

§ 124. For these purposes, every medicinal substance should be employed entirely alone, and in a perfectly pure state, without the admixture of any other substance; and the experimenter (prover) should not partake of any other medicinal substance on the same day. The same caution is to be observed for as many days as the observation of the effects of the drug requires.

§ 125. During the time devoted to the experiment, the diet should be very moderate, as free as possible from spices, and of a simple nutritious kind. Thus, it is advisable to avoid all green vegetables,[93] roots, and all kinds of salad and pot-herbs, all of which retain some disturbing medicinal properties, even if most carefully prepared. Common beverages, not of a stimulating kind,[94] should be used.

§ 126. During the observation of the effect of drugs, the experimenter must avoid mental and bodily exertions, and particularly the disturbances that would result from the excitement of sensual excesses. Nor should experimenters be interrupted in their observations, by urgent business affairs which prevent them from paying close attention to themselves, through fear of disturbance; and, besides being to all intents and purposes of sound health, they should possess the requisite degree of intelligence, to enable them to define, and to describe their sensations in distinct expressions.

§ 127. Drugs should be proved by males as well as by females, in order to discover what effect is produced with regard to the sex.

§ 128. The most recent experiments have taught that crude medicinal substances, if taken by an experimenter for the purpose of ascertaining their peculiar effects, will not disclose the same wealth of latent powers, as when they are taken in a highly attenuated state, potentiated by means of trituration and succussion. Through this simple process the powers bidden and dormant, as it were, in the crude drug, are developed, and called into activity in an incredible degree. In this way, the medicinal powers, even of substances hitherto considered as inert, are most effectually developed by administering to the experimenter daily from four to six of the finest pellets of the thirtieth potentiated attenuation of one of these substances; the pellets having been previously moistened with a little water, should be taken on an empty stomach for several days.

§ 129. If only slight effects appear after a dose of this kind, and if it is desirable to render these effects stronger and more distinct, several additional pellets may be taken daily, until the effects upon the health of the prover become perceptible. A drug does not exert equal strength upon all persons, and a great difference is observable in this respect; for instance, a moderate dose of a drug, known to be very powerful, may sometimes produce but a very slight effect upon an apparently delicate person, while the same individual is affected quite perceptibly by other, much less powerful drugs. Again, there are very robust persons who perceive very marked symptoms from an apparently mild drug, but very slight symptoms from a stronger one. As this is not to be predetermined, it is advisable, that each person should begin with a small dose of medicine, gradually to be increased day by day where such a course appears proper and desirable.

§ 130. By giving a sufficiently strong dose in the beginning of an experiment, we gain the advantage of exhibiting to the experimenter the exact, consecutive order in which the symptoms appear, and of allowing the observer to note the time at which each one appeared. This method proves to be very instructive with regard to the character (genius) of the drug, since it shows most distinctly the order in which primary and secondary effects appear. A moderate dose frequently suffices for the experiment, provided the experimenter is sufficiently sensitive, and pays proper attention to the state of his feelings. The duration of the effect of a drug is determined only after comparison of a number of experiments.

§ 131. But if, in trying to obtain even a slight effect, it becomes necessary to administer increased doses of some drug to a person for several days in succession, we may discover the various morbid conditions which this drug is capable of producing in general; but we will not learn the consecutive order of their appearance, and besides, a second dose, by its curative effect, will often remove some of the symptoms resulting from the previous dose; or a second dose may produce the opposite condition from that of the first. Too frequent a repetition of the dose produces ambiguous symptoms which should be marked as unreliable by inclosing them in brackets, until other, more exact (purer) experiments shall have proved them to be either effect and after-effect of the organism, or alternating effect of the drug.

§ 132. But if it is our purpose to observe a drug of moderate strength, with regard to its symptoms alone, without reference to the consecutive order or duration of the drug-effect, it is preferable to proceed by administering an increased dose for several successive days. In this manner, the effect of every drug, though very mild, and previously unknown, will be disclosed, particularly if it is tested by sensitive persons.

§ 133. When some of the drug-symptoms begin to appear, it is useful and desirable, in order to determine the symptom accurately, that the experimenter assumes various postures, in order to observe if the sensation is increased, lessened, or made to vanish by motion of the affected part; by walking in the room, or in the open air; by standing, sitting, or lying; or whether it returns when he assumes the original position. He should also observe if the symptom is changed by eating, drinking, talking, coughing, sneezing, or some other bodily function. Particular notice should also be taken of the time of the day or night at which each symptom usually appears, in order to discover its peculiarities and characteristics.

§ 134. All noxious agents, and especially drugs, possess the property of producing a particular kind of change in the health of the living organism. But not every symptom peculiar to one drug, appears in the same person; neither do all become manifest at once, nor during a single experiment. A prover first experiences certain symptoms, and others during a second, and a third trial. Other persons may perceive certain symptoms of another kind; while perhaps the fourth, eighth, or tenth experimenter experiences several, or many of the same symptoms which had already been perceived by the second, sixth, or ninth person; neither do these symptoms appear at the same hour.

§ 135. The totality of all the elements of disease which a drug is capable of producing, is brought near perfection only by manifold experiments, instituted by a select variety of individuals of both sexes. We should not consider the proving of a drug as complete, with regard to the morbid conditions it is capable of exciting by means of its peculiar (pure) powers of changing the state of health, until all provers, after repeated trials, cease to perceive new symptoms from the drug, and until they begin to observe, upon themselves, mostly symptoms like those already experienced by others.

§ 136. (As above stated, no drug can produce every variety of symptoms while being proved upon a single, healthy person; it will exhibit this variety only when tested upon many different persons of various bodily and mental constitutions. Nevertheless, the drug possesses the inclination (tendency) to excite all of these symptoms in every person (§ 110). This is founded on an immutable law of nature, in obedience to which, the drug brings into play all its effects, even those rarely produced in the healthy, whenever it is administered to a person suffering from a similar morbid condition. When homœopathically selected, and prescribed even in the mildest dose, it will imperceptibly create in the patient an artificial condition, bearing a very close resemblance to that of the natural disease, and will speedily and permanently cure the sufferer of his original complaints.)

§ 137. Within certain limits of quantity, the smaller the doses are of the drug selected for the purpose of experiment, so much the more distinctly will the primary effects appear which we are most desirous to ascertain. They will appear alone, and without after- or counter-effects of the vital force, provided that observation is facilitated by choosing provers of truthful, temperate habits, of fine powers of perception, and capable of directing close attention to themselves. Excessive doses, on the other hand, cause the result to be disturbed by the appearance of various after-effects among the symptoms, because the primary effects are confused by the haste and violence of the action of the dose, which, besides preventing accurate observation of the effect, causes a certain degree of danger to the prover; this is not considered as a matter of indifference by him who respects the welfare of his fellow-men, and who esteems as his brother the humblest of men.

§ 138. Supposing the above condition, necessary to insure the success and reliability of an experiment, to have been complied with (see §§ 124–127), every symptom, and deviation from the normal state of health, observed by the prover while under the influence of the drug, is derived only from the latter, and must be regarded and noted as a symptom properly belonging to it, notwithstanding the prover may have observed similar and spontaneous sensations upon himself, *some time ago*. The reappearance of the same kind of sensations during the proving of a drug, shows the prover to be particularly susceptible to the influence of drugs, owing to his peculiar bodily constitution. In the present instance, the effect should be ascribed to the drug; for symptoms do not come of themselves; but they are due to the active drug which has been administered, and which controls the state of feeling of the entire organism.

§ 139. If the physician has not taken the drug himself for the purpose of experiment, but has administered it to another person, the latter should distinctly write down every sensation, and change of feeling which he experiences at the time of its occurrence. The time which had elapsed between the taking of the drug, and the appearance of the symptom, should also be noted, as well as the duration of the latter, if it is found possible to do so. The physician should examine the report immediately after the termination of the experiment; or, if this had been extended over several days, the report should be examined daily in the presence of the prover, who should be questioned about the exact form of every symptom while it is yet fresh in his memory; whereupon the information thus obtained concerning particulars, is added to the report, or this may be altered according to subsequent statements.[95]

§ 140. If the prover is not skilled in writing, the physician should inquire every day concerning the nature of symptoms, and the manner of their appearance, in regard to which he should obtain, as far as possible, the voluntary statement of the person employed in the experiment. Whatever is noted in writing as an actual fact, should not consist of guesswork, suppositions, or of extorted statements. This precaution should be strictly observed in every case, as I have explained above (§§ 84–99), while speaking of the manner of exploring natural diseases, and of the precautions to be taken in delineating their true image.

§ 141. The most desirable provings are those which the healthy, unprejudiced physician of fine perception, has made upon himself, for the purpose of discovering the genuine effects which simple drugs may produce in the form of changes of feeling, artificial morbid conditions, and symptoms; and when the physician himself carefully takes every precaution heretofore pointed out, he will be quite sure of what he has observed upon himself.[96]

§ 142. Among the symptoms, especially of chronic diseases, varying little in form, it is sometimes possible to distinguish certain symptoms[97] resulting from a simple drug administered for curative purposes. But this is a matter attended with great difficulty and uncertainty, and should be left only to experts in the art of observing.

§ 143. After a considerable number of simple drugs has been tested in this manner by healthy provers, and after every element, or symptom of disease which these drugs (as artificial morbific agents) are by themselves capable of producing, have been carefully and faithfully recorded, we shall then possess a true Materia Medica. It will consist of a collection of genuine, pure, and undeceptive[98] effects of simple drugs; and will be a code of nature, containing complete records of the particular effects upon health, and the symptoms of every active drug that has been tested, just as they were perceived by the attentive observer. These records will contain, and represent in similitude the (homœopathic) elements of numerous, natural diseases hereafter to be cured by these means. In other words, these records will contain lists of symptoms of artificial diseases; and these afford the only true homœopathic, or specific means for the certain and permanent cure of similar, natural diseases.

§ 144. A Materia Medica of that kind should exclude every supposition, every mere assertion and fiction; its entire contents should be the pure language of nature, uttered in response to careful and faithful inquiry.

§ 145. It is requisite, however, that we should have a large supply of drugs, accurately known with regard to their effects upon the health of the human system, in order to enable us to find[99] a homœopathic remedy, *i. e.*, a suitable analogue, in the form of an artificial morbific (curative) agent for *each* of the countless, morbid conditions in nature,—for *every* disease in the world. But owing to the reliability and wealth of symptoms, or disease-elements which have already been disclosed by observation of the effects of active, medicinal substances upon healthy persons, there remain but few diseases for which suitable homœopathic remedies might not be found among the drugs already tested for their pure effects.[100] By means of such a remedy, health will be restored gently, surely, and permanently, and with far greater certainty and safety than by the general and special therapeutics of the allopathic school, with its compounds of unknown medicines. These only alter and aggravate chronic diseases without curing them, and retard more than they accelerate the recovery from acute diseases.

§ 146. Next to testing drugs for their actual effects on healthy persons, the third portion of the duty of a true physician relates to the homœopathic application of these artificial, morbific potencies (*medicines*), *for the purpose of curing natural diseases.*

§ 147. A drug, completely tested with regard to its power of altering human health, and whose symptoms present the greatest degree of similitude with the totality of symptoms of a given natural disease, will be the most suitable and reliable homœopathic remedy for that disease, for which the specific, curative agent will have been discovered.

§ 148. A medicine possessing the power and inclination to produce similar symptoms, or an artificial disease most similar to the natural disease to be cured, exerts its dynamic influence upon the morbidly disturbed vital force; and if it is administered in well-proportioned dose, it will affect those parts of the organism where the natural disease is located, and will excite in them an artificial disease; this, by virtue of its great similitude and increased intensity, will now occupy the place hitherto held by the natural morbid process. Thereupon the instinctive and automatic vital power is liberated from the natural disease, and is occupied alone with the stronger and similar drug disease. But owing to the minuteness of the dose, this drug affection is sufficiently tractable to allow itself to be overcome by the increased energy of the vital force, and will, therefore, soon vanish, leaving the body free from disease and permanently healthy.

§ 149. If the suitable homœopathic drug is properly selected[101] and applied in this way, a natural, acute disease of recent origin, even if severe and painful, will gently vanish in a few hours; an affection of somewhat older date will disappear in a few days with every trace of discomfort, while little or no effect of the drug will be perceived, and recovery progresses in rapid, though imperceptible stages to the full restoration of health. Old, and particularly complicated diseases demand a greater proportion of time to be cured. Chronic drug diseases, in particular, often complicated in the course of allopathic treatment with an uncured natural disease, yield only after great length of time, if they have not become quite incurable, owing to the wanton waste of strength and substance of the patient; a result very often to be met with after old-school treatment.

§ 150. Whenever a patient complains of only a few insignificant symptoms of very recent origin, the physician is not to regard them as a disease requiring serious medical aid. A slight change of diet, and habits of living, generally suffices to remove so slight an indisposition.

§ 151. But if the symptoms complained of are very severe, though few in number, the physician will, on further inquiry, generally discover several collateral symptoms of less severity, which will serve to complete the picture of the disease.

§ 152. If an acute disease is very severe, the symptoms of which it is composed, will be so much the more conspicuous and numerous, and will increase the certainty of discovering the suitable remedy, provided we possess a sufficient number of medicines whose positive effects are well determined and recorded. From complete catalogues of this kind, it is not difficult to select a remedy out of the individual symptoms of which, we may construe the antitype (Gegenbild) in the form of a curative, artificial disease, very similar to the totality of symptoms of the natural disease; and the medicine exhibiting these symptoms, is the remedy we were in need of.

§ 153. This search for a homœopathic, specific remedy, consists in the *comparison* of the totality of the symptoms of the natural disease with the lists of symptoms of our tested. drugs, among which a morbific potency is to be found, corresponding in similitude with the disease to be cured. In making this comparison, the more *prominent*, *uncommon*, and *peculiar* (characteristic) features of the case[102] are especially, and almost exclusively considered and noted; for *these, in particular, should bear the closest similitude to the symptoms of the desired medicine,* if that is to accomplish the cure. The more general and indefinite symptoms, such as want of appetite, headache, weakness, restless sleep, distress, etc., unless more clearly defined, deserve but little notice on account of their vagueness, and also because generalities of this kind are common to every disease, and to almost every drug.

§ 154. Now, if the antitype, construed out of the symptoms of the most suitable medicine, consists of prominent, uncommon, and characteristic symptoms, equal in number and similitude to the disease to be cured, this *medicine* will prove to be the most homœopathic and specific remedy for the case. A disease of recent date will usually be cancelled and extinguished, without additional discomfort, by the first dose of the remedy.

§ 155. I say, *without additional discomfort.* For, during the action of a homœopathic medicine, only those of its symptoms which correspond to those of the disease, are in active operation; the former occupy the place of the weaker symptoms of the disease; these are thereby extinguished; while the numerous, remaining symptoms of the homœopathic medicine have no affinity to the case, and therefore remain entirely quiescent. Scarcely anything is perceived of them during the gradual progress of improvement, because the minute dose, required in homœopathic practice, is much too weak to allow the non-homœopathic portion of its symptoms visibly to affect the sound parts of the body; therefore only the homœopathic symptoms are permitted to operate upon the parts of the organism which are most decidedly under the influence of the disease, and in this way the diseased vital force is altered by the stronger drug disease in such a manner, that the original disease is extinguished.*

§ 156. There is, however, scarcely a homœopathic remedy which, though well selected, if not sufficiently reduced in its dose, might not call forth at least one unusual sensation, or slight new symptom during its operation on very susceptible and sensitive patients; for it is almost impossible that medicine and disease should possess the same congruity as two triangles of like angles and sides. But this insignificant difference is easily erased by the active energy of the living organism, and is not even perceived by patients of ordinary sensibility. Convalescence will, nevertheless, progress to final recovery, provided it is not interrupted by extraneous medicinal influences, dietetic excesses, or excitement.

§ 157. Although a homœopathically selected remedy, by virtue of its fitness and minuteness of dose, quietly cancels or extinguishes an analogous disease, without manifesting any of its unhomœopathic symptoms; that is to say, without exciting additional, perceptible sensations, it will, nevertheless, as a rule (or in the course of a few hours) produce a slight aggravation resembling the original disease so closely, that the patient actually considers it as such. Aggravation caused by larger doses may last for several hours, but in reality these are only *drug-effects* somewhat superior in intensity, and very similar to the original disease.

---

* As the words "*stronger drug disease,*" implying a curative power, appear somewhat paradoxical, the closing sentence of this paragraph would be more intelligibly rendered thus: . . . . In this way the disturbed vital force is *reinforced by the drug-effect* to such an extent that the original disease is extinguished.—TRANSLATOR.

§ 158. This slight homœopathic aggravation during the first hours, is quite in order, and in case of an acute disease, generally serves as an excellent indication that it will yield to the first dose. The drug-disease must naturally be somewhat more intense in order to overcome and extinguish the natural diseases; as it is only by superior intensity that one natural disease can extinguish another of similar nature (§§ 43–48).

§ 159. The smaller the dose of the homœopathic remedy, so much the smaller and shorter is the apparent aggravation of the disease during the first hours.

§ 160. The dose of a homœopathic remedy can scarcely be reduced to such a degree of minuteness as to make it powerless to overcome, and to completely cure an analogous, natural disease of recent origin, and undisturbed by injudicious treatment (§ 249, remark). We may, therefore, readily understand why a less minute dose of a suitable homœopathic medicine, an hour after its exhibition, may produce an appreciable, homœopathic aggravation of this kind.[103]

§ 161. In stating that the so-called homœopathic aggravation (or, more properly speaking, the primary effect of the homœopathic remedy, which seemingly intensifies the symptoms of the original disease) is liable to occur in the first hours, this is to be understood as referring to acute diseases of recent origin;[104] but whenever medicines of protracted effect, are prescribed in diseases of long standing, where one dose must necessarily extend its operation over many days, such primary drug-effects, resembling an intensification of symptoms of the original disease (lasting an hour or more), will be seen occasionally in the course of six, eight, or ten days, while a general improvement becomes visible in the intervening hours. After the days of aggravation have passed, the convalescence, induced by these primary drug-effects, will progress almost uninterruptedly for several days.

§ 162. As long as we have at our disposal only a limited number of drugs whose actual effects are wholly known, it sometimes occurs that only a portion of the symptoms of the disease we wish to cure, corresponds with those of the medicine selected as the most similar one; we may, therefore, be obliged to resort to a less perfect curative agent, for want of a better one.

§ 163. In this case, a perfect and easy cure cannot be expected to result from the medicine; because disturbances will be observed to follow its use, which were not previously encountered in the disease; these disturbances should be regarded as accessory symptoms of the medicine, imperfectly adapted to the case. But these will not prevent the medicine from obliterating a considerable portion of the disease (*i. e.*, of those disease-symptoms which are similar to the drug-symptoms), thereby making a fair beginning in convalescence; still this will not proceed without accessory effects, which, however, are always moderate, if the dose is sufficiently attenuated.

§ 164. The cure, however, will not be essentially retarded by the scarcity of similar drug-symptoms, provided the remedy is carefully selected, and the symptoms which *determine its choice are mostly peculiar to the remedy, and of marked similitude* (characteristic) *to those of the disease;* in which case, the cure will result without particular inconvenience.

§ 165. But if the case presents no marked and peculiar symptoms of accurate similitude to those of a chosen remedy; and if the latter corresponds to the disease merely in regard to its general and vaguely defined symptoms (such as nausea, weakness, headache, etc.), and if no medicine of close homœopathic relation to the case can be found, the physician will look in vain for an immediate favorable result from the use of this unhomœopathic remedy.

§ 166. Instances of this kind, however, will be *very rare,* owing to the great recent addition of medicines, well tested with reference to their pure effects; and if such a case should occur, the temporary delay in its cure will be removed as soon as a subsequent medicine of more striking similitude is selected.

§ 167. If, in an acute case, accessory disturbances of some importance should result from the first and imperfect homœopathic medicine, its first dose should not be allowed to complete its operation, nor should the patient be left to suffer the entire duration of the effect of the medicine; but his case with its recent changes should now be reexamined, and the remaining original symptoms considered in connection with the accessory ones, for the purpose of construing a new picture of the disease.

§ 168. This will greatly diminish the difficulty of selecting from our stock of well-known medicines, a remedy analogous to the newly examined case; and a single prescription of the remedy will suffice for the cure of the disease, or at least to bring it much nearer to its termination. If this remedy, also, should be found insufficient for the re-establishment of perfect health, the examination of the remaining morbid condition, and the selection of the most suitable homœopathic remedy, should be repeated until the object of restoring the patient to perfect health is accomplished.

§ 169. On account of the limited number of thoroughly known remedies, cases may occur where the first examination of the disease, and the first selection of a remedy prove that the totality of symptoms of the disease is not sufficiently covered by the morbific elements (symptoms) of a single remedy; and where we are obliged to choose between two medicines which seem to be equally well suited to the case, and one of which appears to be homœopathic to a certain portion of the symptoms of the case, while the second is indicated by the other portion. In these instances, after having decided upon, and prescribed one of these medicines as most eligible, it is not advisable to administer the remedy of our second choice without farther scrutiny, because it may no longer correspond to the symptoms which remain after the case has undergone a change. It will, therefore, be our best plan to make a new record of the case, and to find the most homœopathic remedy for the state of the symptoms.

§ 170. In this, as well as in every other case where a change of symptoms has occurred, a new record should be made of the remaining symptoms, and a new homœopathic remedy selected (without regard to that second medicine, which at first appeared as second best), which is adapted as accurately as possible to the new state of the disease as now presented. But if it should appear, as it rarely does, that the medicine of our second choice were still suited to the remnant of the morbid condition, it would now deserve much more confidence, and should be employed in preference to others.

§ 171. In non-venereal chronic diseases, which originated from psora, it is often necessary to employ several antipsoric remedies in succession; each of which in its turn had been homœopathically selected, in accordance with the group of symptoms left uncured when the preceding remedy (given in single, or in repeated doses) had terminated its action.

§ 172. Another embarrassment in the performance of a cure, may arise from the scarcity of symptoms presented by the disease. This is an impediment which merits careful consideration, because its removal will also do away with the most serious difficulties encountered in this perfect method of curing; if we except those arising from the incompleteness of our apparatus of known homœopathic medicines.

§ 173. Diseases which seem to present an insufficient number of symptoms, and which, therefore, appear to be less susceptible of cure, may with propriety be termed *partial* (one-sided) diseases. They present only one or two prominent symptoms, which obscure the remaining features of the case almost entirely. The greater part of such diseases are chronic.

§ 174. Their chief symptoms may indicate either an internal affection, *e. g.*, headache, diarrhœa, or cardialgia of long standing, etc., or it may belong to an affection of more external character. The last-named kind is commonly known as *local* diseases.

§ 175. If in partial diseases of the internal variety, all the symptoms necessary for the completion of the outlines of the case are not entirely discovered, the error is generally to be ascribed to want of attention on the part of the physician.

§ 176. There are, however, a few diseases which, notwithstanding careful investigation at the outset (§§ 84–98), exhibit their peculiarities but imperfectly, with the exception of a few strongly marked and violent symptoms.

§ 177. Rare as these cases may be, we may meet them successfully by making the best use of these few prominent symptoms, which will serve as guides in the selection of a homœopathic remedy.

§ 178. It may certainly happen sometimes, that a medicine selected with careful observance of the homœopathic law, may embrace in its symptoms the similar, artificial disease which is capable of curing the natural partial disease. The possibility of such a result is increased, if the few symptoms of the natural disease are especially peculiar to it, and well defined (characteristic).

§ 179. In most cases, however, the first selected remedy will only be partially, that is, inaccurately adapted, because a proper selection could not be made in the absence of a majority of striking symptoms.

§ 180. Although the homœopathic medicine may have been selected as well as the symptoms of the case would allow, it may be only partially analogous to the disease, and will, therefore, excite accessory symptoms in the same manner, as (§ 162, and the following) where the scarcity of remedies renders their homœopathic adaptation imperfect. An imperfectly adapted remedy will mingle some of its own peculiar symptoms with the feelings of the patient; but they should be regarded as symptoms of the disease itself, although they had rarely or never been perceived before. In other words, sensations will be developed in a higher degree, which the patient had not previously perceived at all, or only imperfectly.

§ 181. The newly presented accessory sensations and symptoms of such a case ought not to be ascribed to the last remedy alone. It is true that they proceed partly from the remedy;[105] but the symptoms are always of a kind which this medicine is of itself capable of producing in a certain kind of constitution, and which are only brought to light by the medicine, as an agent capable of giving rise to similar symptoms. Therefore, the now visible totality of symptoms must be regarded, and consequently treated as belonging to the disease itself, and, in fact, as its true representative condition.

§ 182. Although the remedy may be imperfectly adapted on account of the unavoidable deficiency of symptoms presented by the case, it will, nevertheless, serve the purpose of bringing to light the symptoms belonging to the disease; thus facilitating the task of searching out a second, and more accurately suited homœopathic medicine.

§ 183. As soon, therefore, as the dose of the first medicine ceases its beneficial action, a new record of the disease is to be made, the *status morbi*, as it is, noted, and a new and accurate homœopathic remedy chosen accordingly. This will be readily found, now that the group of symptoms has become more numerous and complete;[106] and it should be administered at once, provided the new symptoms are not sufficiently severe to require more prompt relief; an aggravation of this kind, however, is rarely produced by minute homœopathic doses in diseases of long standing.

§ 184. After the completion of the effect of each dose of medicine, the case should be re-examined, in order to ascertain what symptoms remain; and again a most suitable homœopathic remedy should be selected, corresponding to this newly found group of symptoms; and so on, till health is restored.

§ 185. The so-called local affections occupy a prominent place among partial diseases. The term is applied to diseased conditions appearing upon external parts of the body, which, as the old school teaches, are diseased independently and without the participation of the rest of the body—an absurd theory, that has led, and still leads to the most pernicious treatment.

§ 186. The name of local diseases seems most applicable to those affections which are of recent origin, and caused by external injury. But in that case the injury must have been trifling, and, hence, of no particular significance, because the entire body is made to participate in the suffering caused by external injuries even of moderate severity; as, for instance, when they are followed by febrile conditions. Affections of external parts requiring mechanical skill, properly belong to surgery alone; as, for instance, when external impediments are to be removed that prevent the vital force from accomplishing the cure. Examples of this kind are: reduction of dislocations; the union of edges of wounds by bandages; the extraction of foreign bodies that have penetrated parts of the body; the opening of cavities, either for the removal of cumbersome substances, or to form an outlet to effusions; the approximation of fractured ends of bones, and the retention of the adjusted parts by proper bandages, etc. But frequently the entire organism is affected to such an extent by injuries as to require dynamic treatment, in order that it may be placed in the proper condition for the performance of the curative operation. Where, for instance, an active fever produced by severe contusions, lacerations of muscles, tendons, and vessels is to be subdued by internal administration of medicines, or where the external pain of burnt or corroded parts is to be removed, there the dynamic effect of homœopathic treatment is imperatively called for.

§ 187. But affections of external parts, which are not caused by external injuries, or of which slight injuries may have been only the remote cause, have a source of very different nature, and proceed from an internal morbid state. To designate such conditions merely as local diseases, and to treat them surgically, as it were, and almost exclusively by local applications according to the most ancient custom of medicine, is as absurd as its consequences are disastrous.

§ 188. These evils were simply considered and designated as local affections of separate visible parts upon which they were supposed to occur exclusively, while the rest of the general organism was supposed to take little or no part in them, and to remain unconscious, as it were, of their existence.[107]

§ 189. It becomes apparent upon reflection that no external disease (not occasioned by some particular external lesion) can be originated, hold its place, or, least of all, become aggravated without some internal cause, or without the participation of the organism which, consequently, must share in the morbid condition. An external disease of that kind could never make its appearance without involving the entire state of health, and without the participation of the living whole; that is, of the vital force governing all the other sensitive and irritable parts of the organism. The growth of such a disorder is inconceivable unless called forth by a morbid condition of the entire vital principle. In fact, all parts of the organism are so intimately connected as to form an indivisible whole in feelings and functions, that not even an eruption on the lips, or a case of paronychia can be accounted for without assuming a previous and simultaneous diseased state of the body.

§ 190. In order to combine both safety and thoroughness in the medical treatment of external diseases not dependent upon external lesions, all curative measures should be planned with reference to the state of the *whole system,* in order to effect the obliteration and cure of the general disease by means of internal remedies.

§ 191. This is unequivocally verified by experience, which shows in every instance that each internal active medicine, immediately after having been taken, causes significant changes in the general condition of the patient, and principally also in diseased external and remote parts which are, by the old school, considered as isolated. In fact, a medicine produces the most salutary change in the form of convalescence of the entire body, during which the external evil is seen to disappear without the aid of external medication, provided the internal homœopathic remedy had been properly selected to meet the whole case.

§ 192. This is done most effectually by conducting the examination of a case in such a manner, that the record of the exact state of the *local disease* is added to the summary of all symptoms, and other peculiarities to be observed in the *general condition* of the patient (before, during, and after the use of medicines), in order to complete the record or picture of the disease before proceeding to select (from among the medicines tested with regard to their morbific effects) a homœopathic remedy corresponding to this totality of symptoms.

§ 193. By this internal remedy the general morbid condition of the body is cured simultaneously with the local disease, and sometimes the first dose of the remedy accomplishes this end, if the disease is of recent origin. This proves that the local evil must have depended entirely upon a diseased state of the system in general, and that it was to be regarded as an inseparable part, and as one of the greatest and most prominent symptoms of the entire disease.

§ 194. It is neither beneficial in acute local diseases of rapid growth, nor in those of long standing, to use a remedy externally as a local application to the diseased part, even if the medicines were specific and curative in that form. Acute local diseases, such as inflammations of single parts, like erysipelas, for instance, which are not produced by violent external injuries, but by dynamic or internal causes, will usually yield rapidly to internal homœopathic remedies selected from our stock of well-tested medicines,[108] and adapted to actually perceptible external and internal symptoms. But notwithstanding the well-regulated habits of the patient, a remnant of disease may still be left in the affected part or in the system at large, which the vital force is unable to restore to its normal state; in that case the acute local disease frequently proves to be a product of psora, which has lain dormant in the system, where it is now about to become developed into an actual chronic disease.

§ 195. Causes of this kind are by no means uncommon; and in order to accomplish a thorough cure after the acute condition has been reduced as far as possible, a proper course of antipsoric treatment should be instituted to remove the remainder of the disease, and, at the same time, to relieve the habitual symptoms peculiar to the patient previous to the acute attack (according to the directions given in the book on chronic diseases). The antipsoric, internal treatment is requisite in non-venereal chronic disorders.

§ 196. It may seem as if the cure of a local disease could be accelerated, not only by internal administration, but also by external application of the correct homœopathic remedy adapted to the totality of symptoms, since the effect of a medicine, applied locally to the disease itself, might possibly produce a more rapid improvement.

§ 197. But this kind of treatment is entirely objectionable, not only in local affections dependent on psora, but also in local symptoms arising from syphilis and from sycosis, *because the local application of a medicine, simultaneously with its internal use, results in great disadvan-*

tages. For in diseases characterized by a main symptom in the form of a permanent local affection,[109] the latter is generally dispelled by topical applications more rapidly than the internal disease. This often leads to the deceptive impression that we have accomplished a perfect cure. At all events the premature disappearance of this local symptom renders it very difficult, and in some cases impossible to determine whether the total disease has also been exterminated by the internal remedy.

§ 198. For the same reason, a medicine having the power of curing internally, should not be employed *exclusively as a topical application* to the local symptoms of chronic miasmatic diseases. For, if these are only topically suppressed, this partial effect will leave us in doubt regarding the action of the internal remedies, which are absolutely indispensable to the restoration of general health. The main symptom (local disease) has disappeared, and only the less important symptoms are left; these are so much less constant and reliable than the local disease, and their peculiarities and characteristics are often so indistinct, that they fail to furnish a clear and perfect outline of the disease.

§ 199. Now, if in addition to this, the appropriate homœopathic remedy for the disease[110] has not been found up to the time when the local symptom was obliterated by caustics, escharotics, or by excision, the case will be involved in still greater difficulty, on account of the obscurity and inconstancy of the remaining symptoms. After the external and principal symptom has been placed beyond the reach of our observation, we are deprived of that feature of the case which would have determined the selection of a homœopathic remedy, the internal use of which, could alone have secured complete recovery.

§ 200. If this main symptom were still present, the homœopathic remedy for the whole disease could have been found, and in that case the persistence of the local disease, during the internal operation of the medicine, would prove the incompleteness of the cure. But if the local disease disappears from its site, we would gain an inestimable advantage, and have established evidence of the achievement of a radical cure, and of complete recovery from the general disease.

§ 201. When the system is affected with some chronic disease which threatens to destroy vital organs and life itself, and which does not yield to the spontaneous efforts of the vital force, this endeavors to quiet the inner disease, and to avert the danger by substituting and maintaining a local disease on some external part of the body, whither the internal disease is transferred by derivation. The presence of the local disease for a time arrests the internal evil, without, however, being able to cure it or to lessen it essentially.[111] Nevertheless, the local disease continues to be a part of the general disease; but it is a part which has become excessively developed *in one direction* by the organic vital force, and transported to a more secure portion of the body, in order to lessen the internal morbid process. To soothe the inner disease by a local affection, is of little benefit to the vital force in its effort to reduce and cure the general disease. For, notwithstanding the efforts of nature, the internal disease increases constantly, while nature is compelled gradually to enlarge and aggravate the local symptom, in order to make it a sufficient substitute for, and to subdue the inner disease. Old ulcers of the leg, and chancres are aggravated and enlarged in proportion to the spontaneous growth of internal syphilis and psora which remain un cured.

§ 202. When an old-school physician, acting under the impression that he is curing the whole disease, destroys the local symptom by external remedies, nature will offset it by awakening and extending the inner disease, and all the dormant symptoms which had previously coexisted with the local affection. A case of this kind is then incorrectly defined in popular phrase, by saying that the topical medicine had driven the whole disease back into the system upon the nerves.

§ 203. Many kinds of external treatment are in vogue for the removal of local symptoms from the surface of the body, without curing the inner miasmatic disease. It is customary, for instance, to remove the itch from the skin by all kinds of ointments; to destroy chancres externally by cauterization; and locally to exterminate sycotic excrescences by excision, ligature, or the actual cautery. This method of external treatment hitherto so common, is pernicious in its results, and is the most general source of innumerable chronic diseases with and without names, under the burden of which the human race suffers; although one of the most culpable habits of the medical profession, it was hitherto generally introduced, and is proclaimed by professors as the only reliable method of practice.[112]

§ 204. By placing into one class all protracted diseases arising from unwholesome habits of living, together with countless drug-diseases (see § 74), produced by the persistent and debilitating treatment often employed by old-school physicians in trifling disorders, we shall then find that all other chronic diseases, without exception, are derived from the development of three chronic miasms: internal syphilis, internal sycosis, but chiefly and in far greater proportion internal psora. Each of these must have pervaded the entire organism, and penetrated all its parts before the primary, representative local symptom, peculiar to each miasm (itch eruption of psora, chancre and bubo of syphilis, and condyloid excrescences of sycosis) makes its appearance for the prevention of the inner disease. When its local symptom is suppressed, the internal disease will be developed sooner or later, in obedience to the laws of nature. It will be followed by endless misery in the form of innumerable chronic diseases which have been the scourge of the human race for thousands of years, and these would never have prevailed to such an extent, had physicians endeavored rationally and zealously to cure and eradicate each miasm by internal homœopathic treatment and well-selected medicines, instead of tampering with their local symptoms by topical applications.

§ 205. Homœopathic practice never requires us to single out some primary or secondary symptom resulting from chronic miasm, nor to resort to external local remedies, either dynamic[113] or mechanical. But wherever one of these symptoms appears, homœopathy cures the great fundamental miasm, together with which its primary as well as its secondary symptoms vanish simultaneously. But as the homœopathic physician will generally find the primary symptoms[114] to have been suppressed by local treatment of allopathic practitioners, it will be his duty to accomplish what his predecessors neglected to do.

He will, therefore, give his attention more particularly to the secondary symptoms which result from the development of an inner miasm, and will observe especially chronic diseases arising from internal psora. I have endeavored to demonstrate the internal treatment of these diseases, as far as it was possible for a single physician to do, after many years of thought, observation, and experience, in my book on chronic diseases, to which I herewith refer the reader.

§ 206. Before beginning the treatment of a chronic disease, it is necessary to inquire most carefully[115] if the patient had been infected by venereal disease, or by sycotic gonorrhœa. In either case the treatment should be directed against the affection whose symptoms are alone found to be present; although it is rare in modern times to meet with uncomplicated cases of these affections. If such an infection is acknowledged by the patient, it should also be taken into consideration when *psora* is the principal object of treatment, because the latter will have been complicated with the former, a condition always indicated when the symptoms of psora are mingled with others. When a physician is called to treat what he supposes to be an inveterate case of syphilis, he will usually find that it is principally complicated with psora, because the inner itch miasm, or psora, *is by far the most frequent and fundamental cause of chronic diseases*, and is frequently complicated either with syphilis or with sycosis, if infection with the latter has taken place. But in by far the majority of cases, psora is the sole and fundamental cause of chronic diseases, whatever their names may be, and these are often exaggerated and distorted by allopathic interference.

§ 207. After these conditions have been fulfilled, it remains for the homœopathic physician to inquire to what allopathic treatment the patient had been hitherto subjected, and what active medicines he had chiefly and most frequently used. It should also be ascertained what mineral baths he had employed, and with what result, in order to understand the deviations which this treatment had produced in the original disease; and to determine the course to be pursued, to correct, if possible, this artificial deterioration, or, at least, to avoid henceforth those medicines which had been abused.

§ 208. Next to this, the patient's age, mode of living and diet, occupation, domestic circumstances, and even his social position are to be considered, in order to see if these have been of a nature to augment the disease, or in what respect the cure might be favored or impeded thereby. Neither should the physician overlook the patient's state of mind and temperament, and observe if it inclines to prevent the cure, or whether it might be necessary to direct or modify his mental condition by psychical means.

§ 209. After these points have received attention according to the above directions, and after several interviews, the physician will find himself enabled to determine the state of the patient's case as perfectly as possible, and to mark the most conspicuous and peculiar (characteristic) symptoms. Guided by these, and in accordance with strict similitude of symptoms, he should then select the first antipsoric, antisyphilitic, or antisycotic remedy for the beginning of the cure.

§ 210. Most diseases which I have previously described

as partial, belong to psora, and these appear to be more difficult to cure owing to this partial development, where all other symptoms of the disease are obscured by the presence of one, great, prominent symptom. The so-called *diseases of the mind and temperament* are of this kind. These, however, do not constitute a class of diseases strictly distinct from others, because the state of the mind is *always modified*[116] in so-called physical diseases; and hence the state of the mind, being one of the most important features of the complex of symptoms, is to be noted, in order to secure a reliable record (picture) of all diseases presenting themselves for treatment, and that each may be effectually and homœopathically cured.

§ 211. The state of the patient's mind and temperament is often of most decisive importance in the homœopathic selection of a remedy, since it is a distinct and peculiar symptom that should least of all escape the accurate observation of the physician.

§ 212. The effect upon the state of mind and disposition is the principal feature of all diseases, and seems to have been specially ordained by the Creator of all healing powers. There is not a single potent medicinal substance that does not possess the power of altering perceptibly the mental condition and mood of a healthy person who voluntarily tests a drug; indeed, each medicinal substance affects the mind in a different manner.

§ 213. The treatment would not be in accordance with nature, that is, homœopathic, unless we recognize also the symptomatic changes of mind and temperament occurring in every case of acute as well as of chronic disease, and unless we select from our remedies one which, next to the similitude of its physical symptoms to those of the disease, is also capable of producing by itself a similar effect upon the mind and disposition.[117]

§ 214. What I have to say regarding the treatment of mental diseases, may be expressed in a few words. Such diseases are to be treated like all others, and they are curable only by means of a remedy which is very similar to the disease, with regard to the morbific effects it is capable of producing upon the bodily and mental state of a healthy person.

§ 215. Most of the so-called diseases of the mind are in reality bodily diseases. Certain mental and emotional symptoms are peculiar to every bodily disease; these symptoms develop more or less rapidly, assume a state of most conspicuous one-sidedness, and are finally transferred, like a local disease, into the invisibly fine organs of the mind, where, by their presence, they seem to obscure the bodily symptoms.

§ 216. It is a common observation that a dangerous physical disease, such as suppuration of the lungs, or other destructive and acute affections (like those following childbirth), have certain mental symptoms. These are subject to rapid development, and often degenerate into insanity, melancholy, or raving madness, whereby all threatening bodily symptoms are made to vanish, and seem to be replaced by perfect health; or, rather, they diminish to such a degree, that their presence, though obscured, is discovered only by the utmost vigilance and care on the part of the physician. In this manner they assume the shape of one-sided, or, as it were, of local diseases which have the peculiarity, that a slight degree of mental disturbance is enlarged into the main symptom, which henceforth serves as a substitute for the rest of the physical symptoms, and palliates their violence. In short, the disorders of the coarser bodily organs are transferred, as it were, to the almost spiritual organs of the mind, where the dissecting-knife will search in vain for their cause.

§ 217. In these diseases the observation of every symptom should be conducted with the utmost care. We should obtain most exact knowledge of the bodily symptoms, particularly also of the definite peculiarity and character of the main feature of the complex of symptoms, *i. e.*, of the precise condition of the mind and disposition prevailing in each case. We shall then be in a position to select from the remedies known according to their actual effects, one that will cure the entire disease. The remedy thus chosen should exhibit symptoms of the greatest similitude, not only to those of the bodily disease, but also to those of the mind and temperament.

§ 218. In recording the totality of symptoms of a case of this kind, it is of prime importance to obtain an accurate description of all physical symptoms which prevailed before the disease degenerated into a one-sided mental disorder. The information necessary for this purpose will be derived from the statements of the attendants of the patient.

§ 219. We may obtain assurance of the continued, though obscured, existence of the physical disease, by comparing its *early symptoms* with their *present indistinct remnants* which occasionally appear during lucid intervals, and during transient amelioration of the mental disease.

§ 220. To complete the record of the totality, it is necessary to add the symptoms of the mental state as observed by the physician and attendants of the patient. We may then proceed to find a remedy of great similitude, especially with regard to the mental disturbance which it has the power to produce; and if the case is a chronic one, its remedy will be found among the antipsorics.

§ 221. Insanity or madness is sometimes occasioned by fright, vexation, spirituous liquors, etc., and takes the form of an acute affection, suddenly interrupting the ordinary quiet course of the disease; and, although it may be traced to latent psora, it would not be advisable to treat this acute attack with antipsoric remedies at once. It should be met at first by well-proved remedies of the other class, such as Aconite, Belladonna, Stramonium, Hyoscyanus, Mercurius, etc., administered in highly attenuated homœopathic doses. These will subdue it so far, that the psora is for the present forced to return to its latent condition, whereupon the patient will appear to have recovered.

§ 222. Although a patient is relieved of an acute mental disorder by means of non-antipsoric medicines, he should not be considered as entirely cured. On the contrary, no time is to be lost in perfecting the cure[118] by means of continued antipsoric treatment, in order to free the patient from the chronic miasm of psora which, though apparently latent, is apt to break out anew. After such treatment, no fear need be entertained of another attack of the same kind, provided the patient will faithfully adhere to well-regulated diet and habits.

§ 223. If the antipsoric treatment is omitted, a new, more protracted, and serious attack of insanity may be called forth by much slighter causes than the first. During this second attack, psora is usually developed, and may assume the form, either of a periodical or a continuous affection of the mind, which is then much more difficult to cure.

§ 224. Mental disease may not be fully developed, or there may be some doubt as to its origin from physical disease, or from educational errors, bad habits, corrupt morals, neglected mental training, superstition, or ignorance. In these cases, the following will serve as means of distinguishing the cause: if the mental affection is based on the last-named class of causes, it will yield and improve under the influence of sensible admonition and consolation, or of serious remonstrances and arguments; while real mental disorders arising from physical disease, are rapidly aggravated by the same measures. Thus, melancholy patients will be still more depressed, plaintive, disconsolate, and retiring; the malicious maniac will be still more embittered; and the silly prattler will become more foolish than ever.[119]

§ 225. There are, nevertheless, some mental diseases which are not the result of physical or bodily affections, but which, notwithstanding tolerably good physical health, originate in, and proceed directly from the mind. They are often caused by protracted grief, mortification, vexation, insult, and frequent occurrence of intense fear, or fright. This kind of mental affection, in the course of time, will also seriously deteriorate the bodily health.

§ 226. When this kind of mental affections, bred and nourished by the soul itself, *are of recent date, and have not yet undermined the physical health too seriously*, they admit of speedy cure by psychical treatment: gentleness, kind admonition, appeals to reason, and often skilful deception, will soon restore health and comfort to the mind, while careful regulation of habits will reëstablish the health of the body also.

§ 227. These diseases are likewise founded on psoric miasm which had not attained its full development. As a measure of precaution, therefore, it is desirable to subject the convalescent patient to a course of thorough antipsoric treatment, in order to prevent a recurrence of the attack of mental aberration which might readily occur.

§ 228. Although diseases of the mind and temperament, of physical origin, are only to be cured by antipsoric homœopathic medicine, combined with carefully regulated habits, it is necessary, also, to unite this treatment with proper hygiene and psychical regimen of the mind, to be strictly enforced by the physician and attendants of the patient. Raving madness should be met by calm fearlessness and firmness of will; painfully plaintive melancholy should be soothed by silent compassion conveyed by gestures and expression of countenance; silly loquacity should be listened to in silence, but with some degree of attention; indecent behavior and obscene language are to be treated with indifference. The destruction and injury of objects should be simply prevented by placing them out of reach, *without reproaching the patient for his conduct;* furthermore, the treatment should be conducted with a view to the absolute avoidance of corporeal punishment or torture.[120] The administration of medicines would alone justify coercion; but this is easily to be avoided on account of the smallness of the dose, and absence of taste of homœopathic medicines. These do not excite suspicion, and may, therefore, be given to the patient, mixed in his usual drink, without his knowledge, thus obviating every kind of compulsion.

§ 229. On the other hand contradiction, incessant argument, violent remonstrance, and vituperation, no less than weak and timid submission, are altogether out of place, and alike hurtful as means of treating diseases of the mind. There is nothing that embitters the insane, and augments their diseases so much, as expressions of contempt, and ill-disguised deception. *The physician and attendant should always treat such patients as if they regarded them as rational beings.*

Therefore every disturbance of the senses and of the mind should be avoided. There is no entertainment to fascinate their benighted spirit; neither words, books, nor other objects will soothe the rebellious soul, now roused to madness, now languishing imprisoned in the body shattered by disease. A perfect cure alone will bring comfort; rest and relief will return to the mind, only when the body is restored to health.

§ 230. For the purpose of cure, antipsoric remedies should be most homœopathically adapted to the carefully recorded symptoms (image) of each individual case of mental disease, whose varieties are innumerable. This adaptation is readily effected by diligent search for a suitable homœopathic remedy, provided we possess a sufficient number of known remedies to choose from. The selection is likewise facilitated by the mental affection in its character as chief symptom of the case, pointing to the remedy with unmistakable clearness. When the remedy is well adapted, the minutest dose often produces a remarkable improvement in a short time, which could not have been attained by the largest and frequent doses of all other inappropriate (allopathic) medicines, even if pushed to the last extreme. Indeed, manifold experiences enable me to assert that the great excellence of homœopathic treatment, compared with all other curative methods, is never more triumphantly exhibited than when applied to chronic mental diseases, which originally sprung from bodily affections, or appeared simultaneously with them.

§ 231. The class of intermittent diseases also claims our special attention. There are those which return at certain periods; and there exists also a great number of intermittent fevers, as well as numerous apparently non-febrile affections resembling the intermittents by their periodical recurrence. Furthermore, there are affections characterized by the appearance of certain morbid conditions, alternating at uncertain periods with morbid conditions of a different kind.

§ 232. The order of *alternating* diseases is also of great variety,[121] but all belong to the class of chronic diseases which are mostly a product of developed psora. In some rare instances they are complicated with syphilitic miasm. In the first instance, they are cured by antipsoric medicines, but in the latter case the treatment should be conducted by alternating antipsorics with antisyphilitics, according to the instructions contained in the book on chronic diseases.

§ 233. *Typical intermittent diseases* are those of a uniform morbid condition which recurs after a certain period of apparent health, and which again vanishes after an equally definite period. This is to be observed in seemingly feverless diseases of intermittent type, as also in a great variety of febrile diseases like intermittent fevers.

§ 234. Apparently non-febrile morbid conditions which recur at stated periods with some patients, are not of sporadic or epidemic nature; but they always belong to the class of chronic, and mostly of genuine psoric diseases. They are rarely combined with syphilis, and if so, they are effectually treated according to the above suggestions. But sometimes an intercurrent dose of potentiated tincture of Peruvian bark is necessary for the purpose of completely extinguishing the intermittent type of these diseases.

§ 235. In sporadic or epidemic intermittents,[122] not prevalent endemically in marshy districts, we often observe that each attack is composed of two distinct stages, such as chill and then heat, or heat and then chill; but still more frequently they consist of three stages, viz., cold, heat, and finally sweat. Hence, the remedy selected for these diseases from the general class of proved medicines (usually the non-antipsorics), should also possess the power of producing in healthy persons, the several successive stages similar to the natural disease. The remedy, in its similitude of symptoms, should correspond as closely as possible with the most prominent and peculiar stage of the disease. It should be homœopathic either to the cold stage and its collateral symptoms, or to the hot stage and its collateral symptoms, according to the most marked peculiarity of these stages. But the symptoms which mark the condition of the patient during the period of intermission, should chiefly be taken as guides in selecting the most striking homœopathic remedy.[123]

§ 236. In these cases, the medicine is generally most efficacious when it is administered a short time after the termination of the paroxysm, when the patient has partially recovered from it. During the intermission the medicine will have time to develop its curative effect in the organism, without violent action or disturbance; while the effect of a medicine, though specifically adapted to the case, given just before the next paroxysm, would coincide with the renewal of the disease, thereby creating such counteraction and distress in the organism, as to deprive the patient of much strength, and even to endanger life.[124] But if the medicine is given just after the termination of the attack, when the fever has entirely subsided, and before the premonitory symptoms of the next paroxysm have time to appear, the vital force of the organism is in the most favorable condition to be gently modified by the medicine, and restored to healthy action

§ 237. If the feverless interval is very brief, as in some severe fevers, or if it is disturbed by the after-effects of the preceding paroxysm, the dose of homœopathic medicine should be administered when the perspiration diminishes, or when the subsequent stages of the paroxysm decline.

§ 238. One dose of the appropriate medicine may prevent several attacks, and may actually have restored health; nevertheless, we may perceive threatening indications of a new attack, and in this case only, the same remedy should be repeated, provided the complex of symptoms continues to be the same. After an interval of health, the recurrence of intermittent fever is possible, only when the noxious influence which first originated the disease, continues to act upon the convalescent patient, as would be the case in marshy localities. Perfect recovery, therefore, can be secured alone by avoiding this exciting cause; that is, by removing the patient to a mountainous region, if the fever occurred in a marshy district.

§ 239. Almost every drug, in its pure effect, produces a specific distinct kind of fever, and even a species of intermittent fever with its alternating stages, differing from fevers produced by other drugs. Therefore nature's bountiful store of medicines will also furnish homœopathic remedies for the numerous natural forms of intermittent fevers. Although the number of medicines tested for their effects upon the healthy is still limited, remedies will be found for many of these fevers.

§ 240. If the homœopathic specific remedy, adapted to the prevalent epidemic of intermittent fevers, should fail in some cases to accomplish a perfect cure, and unless continued exposure to marsh-miasm is at fault, we may conclude that latent psora prevents recovery, and that antipsoric medicines are required to complete the cure.

§ 241. Epidemics of intermittents occurring in places where such fevers are not epidemic, partake of the nature of chronic diseases, and are composed of a series of acute attacks. Each epidemic possesses a peculiar uniform character, common to all individuals attacked by the epidemic disease. By observing the complex of symptoms peculiar to all patients, this common character will be found to point out the homœopathic (specific) remedy for all cases in general. This remedy will also usually relieve patients who, previous to this epidemic, had enjoyed good health, and who were free from developed psora.

§ 242. If in such an epidemic the first attacks befalling an individual, were left uncured, or if the patients had been weakened by allopathic abuses, the latent psora pervading the organism of many, becomes developed, assumes the type of epidemic intermittent fevers, and apparently plays their parts; so that a non-antipsoric medicine which might have been beneficial in the neglected primary attack, is no longer suitable, and utterly useless. In this case we shall have to contend with a psoric intermittent fever, which usually yields only to the finest doses of sulphur and liver of sulphur, repeated at long intervals.

§ 243. A certain malignant form of intermittents, which attack single individuals not residing in marshy localities, are to be treated *in the beginning* like other acute diseases (which, like intermittents, are of psoric origin), by selecting for the special case, a homœopathic remedy from the class of non-antipsoric medicines; this remedy should be continued for several days, for the purpose of reducing the disease as far as possible. But if the disease does not yield to the treatment, we may be assured that psora is in the act of development, and that antipsoric medicines alone will afford perfect relief in the case.

§ 244. Intermittent fevers, which are indigenous to marshy regions, or places subject to inundations, try the patience of the old-school physician; and yet young and healthy persons may become accustomed to marshy regions, and remain healthy if their habits are temperate, and if they are not weakened by want, fatigue, or excesses. Endemic intermittents will attack such persons only as new-comers; but one or two of the smallest doses of highly potentiated Cinchona will easily rid him of the fever, provided his mode of life is simple. However, if persons accustomed to proper physical exercise, and to wholesome bodily and mental habits, are not relieved of marsh intermittents by one or two of such small doses of Cinchona, they are always based upon psora ready to be developed. And hence such persons cannot be cured of intermittents in a marshy region without antipsoric treatment.[125] Occasionally patients of this kind, if they speedily move from a marshy district to a dry, mountainous locality, will apparently recover, provided the disease is not too deeply seated, *i. e.*, if psora is not yet fully developed, so that it might again assume its latent state; such patients, however, will never be restored to perfect health without antipsoric treatment.

§ 245. Now that we have learned the rules to be followed during homœopathic treatment concerning the main differences of diseases, and the particular circumstances attending such diseases, we come to the consideration of *curative remedies*, their mode of application, and the dietetic rules to be observed.

Perceptible and continued progress of improvement in an acute or chronic disease, is a condition which, as long as it lasts, invariably counterindicates the repetition of any medicine whatever, because the beneficial effect which the medicine continues to exert is rapidly approaching its perfection. Under these circumstances every new dose of any medicine, even of the last one that proved beneficial, would disturb the process of recovery.

§ 246. A very fine dose of a well-selected homœopathic remedy, if uninterrupted in its action, will gradually accomplish all of the curative effect it is capable of producing, in a period varying from forty to one hundred days. But it rarely is interrupted, and besides, the physician as well as the patient usually desire to accelerate the cure by reducing this period of time, if possible, by one-half, one-quarter, or even less. Experience has proved in numerous instances that such a result may actually be obtained under the following three conditions: First, by careful selection of the most appropriate homœopathic medicine; secondly, by administering the medicine in the finest dose capable of restoring the vital force to harmonious activity, without causing violent reaction; and, thirdly, by repeating the finest dose of an accurately selected medicine at proper intervals,[126] such as are proved by experience to be most conducive to a speedy cure, and timed so as to prevent an injurious and revulsive counteraction of the vital force, whose action is to be tempered and modified in accordance with the morbific power of the medicine which is similar in effect to the natural disease.

§ 247. Under these conditions the finest doses of the most nicely selected homœopathic medicine may be repeated with excellent, and often astonishing effect, at intervals of fourteen, twelve, ten, eight, or seven days. In chronic diseases assuming an acute form, and demanding greater haste, these spaces of time may be abbreviated still more, but in acute diseases the remedies may be repeated at much shorter intervals; for instance, twenty-four, twelve, eight, or four hours; and in the most acute diseases at intervals varying from an hour to five minutes. These periods are always to be determined by the more or less acute course of the disease, and by the nature of the remedy employed, in accordance with the more definite directions given in the explanatory note to the preceding paragraph.

§ 248. The dose of the same medicine is to be repeated several times if necessary, but only until recovery ensues, or *until the remedy ceases to produce improvement; at that period the remainder of the disease, having suffered a change in its group of symptoms, requires another homœopathic medicine.*

§ 249. Every medicine which, in the course of its operation, produces new and troublesome symptoms not peculiar to the disease to be cured, is incapable of effecting a real improvement,[127] and is not to be considered as homœopathic to the case. If the aggravation produced by this medicine is very perceptible, it should speedily be partially counteracted by an antidote before prescribing the next remedy, which is to be selected with greater care in regard to its similitude to the case. Or, if the accessory symptoms are not too violent, the next remedy should be given at once, in order to replace the inappropriate one.

§ 250. If, in urgent cases the observant physician becomes convinced, after six or twelve hours, that he had been mistaken in the selection of his last remedy, from the fact that the condition of the patient grows worse from hour to hour, as indicated by the appearance of new symptoms, however slight they may be, he will be justified, and in duty bound, to repair his mistake (§ 167) by selecting and administering a homœopathic remedy with greater care, and adapting it more accurately to the new state of the case.

§ 251. There are some medicines (*e. g.*, Ignatia amara, Bryonia, and Rhus rad., and in some respects Belladonna) whose power of affecting the state of health is evinced principally by alternating effects. These are symptoms composed of partly opposite primary effects. If, after the exhibition of one of these remedies, notwithstanding its most careful selection, no improvement is to be observed, this will soon be obtained (in a few hours in acute cases) by a new and equally fine dose of the same remedy.[128]

§ 252. But if it should appear during the use of other medicines that a properly reduced dose of homœopathic (antipsoric) medicine does not produce progressive improvement in a chronic (psoric) disease, it is a certain indication that the cause of the disease still continues to act, and that there is some irregularity of regimen, or some other injurious influence acting upon the patient, which must be removed before a permanent cure can be accomplished.

§ 253. Although not visible to all, the condition of the mind, and the general behavior of the patient are among the most certain and intelligible signs of incipient improvement, or of aggravation in all diseases, especially in acute ones. Incipient improvement, however slight, is indicated by increased sensation of comfort, greater tranquillity and freedom of the mind, heightened courage, and a return of naturalness in the feelings of the patient. The signs of aggravation, however slight they may be, are the opposite of the preceding, and consist in an embarrassed, helpless state of mind, while the deportment, attitude, and actions of the patient appeal to our sympathy. This condition is readily to be seen, or demonstrated to a careful observer, but not to be described in so many words.[129]

§ 254. A physician accustomed to close observation, will experience no great difficulty in distinguishing aggravation from improvement, by the appearance of new symptoms, by an increase of those already present, or by the diminution of the original symptoms undisturbed by new ones, although patients are met with who are incapable of reporting, or disinclined to acknowledge either an improvement or an aggravation.

§ 255. The truth may be ascertained in such cases by examining the patient closely upon every symptom contained in the written record of the case. If these show that neither new and unusual symptoms have appeared, and that none of the old ones have increased, and especially if the state of the mind and disposition is found to be improved, the medicine must have also produced an essential and general improvement of the disease; or, if sufficient time had not been allowed for the action of the medicine, such an improvement may, at all events, soon be expected. But if visible improvement is delayed beyond expectation, supposing the remedy to have been appropriate, the delay should be ascribed to some fault in the regimen of the patient, or to the protracted homœopathic aggravation produced by the medicine (§ 157), and hence the delay must finally be attributed to insufficient reduction of the dose.

§ 256. On the other hand, if the patient mentions some new and important symptoms, this indicates that the medicine had not been homœopathically selected, and though the invalid may kindly assure us that he is improving in health, his statement is not to be implicitly trusted, but his condition is rather to be considered as having undergone a change for the worse, which will soon become quite apparent.

§ 257. A true physician will know how to avoid the habit of considering certain remedies as favorites, merely because he happened to find them frequently adapted to diseases, and followed by favorable results. Such a habit would lead to the neglect of other medicines which, though less frequently applicable, might, nevertheless, be often more homœopathic, and consequently more beneficial.

§ 258. Nor should a physician yield to doubt and weakness so far as to reject those medicines which now and then proved to be inefficacious, owing to improper selection, or because they were unhomœopathic to some particular case of disease. For, in either instance the fault is the physician's, or the supposition a wrong one; he will remember that of all medicines *that* one only deserves attention and preference, which bears accurate similitude to the totality of characteristic symptoms of the case, and that paltry prejudices should never be allowed to interfere with the serious deliberation demanded by the choice of a remedy.

§ 259. The minuteness of the dose required in homœopathic practice, makes it necessary that every other kind of medicinal influence that might cause a disturbance should be avoided in the *diet and regimen* of patients, in order that the highly rarified dose may not be counteracted, overpowered, or disturbed by extraneous medicinal influences.[130]

§ 260. In chronic cases, therefore, it is especially necessary to search carefully for such impediments to the cure, because these diseases are frequently aggravated by obscure noxious influences of that kind, as well as by errors in regimen which, being frequently overlooked, exercise a deleterious effect.[131]

§ 261. The proper regimen to be enjoined during the use of medicines in chronic diseases, consists in the removal of all obstacles in the way of recovery, and in the substitution of a wholesome mode of life, such as innocent recreation of the mind, active exercise in the open air in all kinds of weather (daily walks, light manual labor), proper nutritious food and drink unadulterated with medicinal substances.

§ 262. In acute diseases, on the contrary (insanity excepted) the fine, unerring inner sense of the active instinct of self-preservation will decide the course to be pursued so clearly, that the physician will only have to advise the friends and attendants to obey this voice of nature by gratifying the patient's ardent desires, without offering and urging him to accept hurtful things.

§ 263. The food and drink most commonly craved by patients suffering from acute diseases, is generally of a palliative and soothing kind, and not properly of a medicinal nature, but merely adapted to the gratification of a certain longing. Slight obstacles which moderate gratification might place in the way of recovery,[132] are more than counterbalanced by the power of a homœopathic medicine, by the vital force liberated by the medicine, and by the refreshing effect of a gratified desire. In acute diseases the temperature of the chamber, and the quantity of covering should be regulated entirely according to the wishes of the patient; while every kind of mental exertion, and emotional disturbance is to be carefully avoided.

§ 264. The physician should have at his disposal only *genuine and unadulterated medicines, retaining their full virtues;* in order that he may rely entirely on their curative powers, he should be previously assured of their genuineness.

§ 265. He should most conscientiously assure himself in every instance, that the patient takes the remedy selected for him.

§ 266. Substances derived from the animal and vegetable kingdoms, in their crude state possess the strongest medicinal properties.[133]

§ 267. The active principles of indigenous and freshly

gathered plants, are most perfectly obtained by mixing their expressed juice *at once* with equal parts of strong alcohol. Having waited twenty-four hours for the fibrinous and albuminous matter to subside in the liquid contained in well-stoppered bottles, the clear fluid is decanted and preserved for medicinal use.[134] By the admixture of alcohol, fermentation of vegetable juice is at once arrested, and absolutely prevented for the future, and its medicinal powers are thus preserved without danger of deterioration, for all times, in well-corked bottles, protected from sunlight.[135]

§ 268. Powdered barks, seeds, and roots of foreign plants which cannot be obtained in their fresh condition, should not be used without assurance of their genuineness; this may be ascertained by examining these drugs in their crude and entire state, before making the least medicinal use of them.[136]

§ 269. To serve the purposes of homœopathy, the spiritlike medicinal powers of crude substances are developed to an unparalleled degree by means of a process which was never attempted before, and which causes medicines to penetrate the organism, and thus to become more efficacious and remedial; it is applicable even to those substances which, in their crude state, do not evince the least medicinal effect upon the human body.

§ 270. Thus, two drops of the fresh vegetable juice mixed with an equal proportion of alcohol, are diluted with 98 drops of alcohol, and potentiated by two succussions of the hand; this is the first development of power (potency). The same process is then to be repeated with 29 successive vials, each vial to contain 99 drops of alcohol, filling three-quarters of the vial; this second vial is then to be shaken twice,[137] and so on to the 30th development of power; this is the potentiated decillion-fold dilution ($\overline{X}$), and the one to be commonly used.

§ 271. With the exception of sulphur, which, of late has been used only in the form of highly diluted tincture ($\overline{X}$), all other substances destined for medicinal use, such as pure metals, their oxides or sulphurets, and other minerals; also petroleum, phosphorus, and many animal and vegetable substances, which are only to be obtained in a dried state; neutral salts, etc., are all first to be potentiated to the million-fold dry or powder-dilution, by triturating them for three hours; thereupon, one grain of the trituration is to be dissolved, and diluted in twenty-seven successive vials, up to the 30th potency, or development of power.[138]

§ 272. In the treatment of disease, only one *simple* medicinal substance should be used at a time.[139]

§ 273. It is impossible to conceive why there should be the least doubt as to whether it is more natural and rational to prescribe a single well-known medicine at a time for a disease, or to give a mixture composed of several different medicines.

§ 274. Perfectly simple, unmixed, and single remedies afford the physician all the advantages he could possibly desire. He is enabled to cure natural diseases safely and permanently through the homœopathic affinity of these artificial morbific potencies; and in obedience to the wise maxim that "it is useless to apply a multiplicity of means, where simplicity will accomplish the end," he will never think of giving more than one simple medicine at a time. Even in taking it for granted that all simple medicines were completely proved with regard to their pure and peculiar action upon the healthy human body, the physician would abstain from mixing and compounding drugs, aware that it is impossible to foresee the variety of effects, that two or more medicines, contained in a mixture, might have; or how one might modify and counteract the effect of the other, when introduced into the human body. It is equally certain, on the other hand, that a simple medicine, well selected, will by itself, be quite sufficient to give relief in diseases whereof the totality of symptoms is accurately known. Supposing, even, that a medicine had not been selected quite in accordance with the similitude of symptoms, and that, consequently, it did not alleviate the disease, it would nevertheless be useful by adding to our knowledge of curative remedies. By calling forth new symptoms in such a case, the medicine might corroborate those symptoms which it had already manifested in experiments upon healthy persons—an advantage which is not to be gained by the use of compound medicines.[140]

§ 275. The fitness of a medicine in a given case of disease, does not depend alone upon its accurate homœopathic selection, but also upon the requisite and proper size, or rather minuteness of the dose. *Too strong* a dose of medicine, though quite homœopathic, notwithstanding its remedial nature, will necessarily produce an injurious effect. Its quantity, as well as its homœopathic similitude, will produce an unnecessary surplus of effect upon the over-excited vital force; which, in its turn, acts upon the most sensitive portions of the organism, already most seriously affected by the natural disease.

§ 276. For this reason, too large a dose of medicine, though homœopathic to the case, will be injurious; not only in direct proportion to the largeness of the dose, but also in proportion to its homœopathic similitude, and to the degree of potentiation of the medicine;[141] and it will prove to be far more injurious than an equally large dose of unhomœopathic medicine in every respect unsuited (allopathic) to the disease. In that case, the so-called homœopathic aggravation (*i. e.*, the artificial and similar drug-disease, called forth in the diseased parts of the body by the excessive dose, and the reacting vital force, §§ 157–160), will rise to an injurious height;[142] while the same similar drug-disease, *if excited within proper limits*, would have gently effected a cure. Although the patient will no longer suffer from the original disease which had been homœopathically cured, yet he will have to endure the exaggerated drug-disease, and unnecessary loss of strength.

§ 277. For these reasons, and also because a medicine is of great efficacy when it is quite homœopathic to the case, its curative power will be wonderfully increased in proportion to the reduction of the dose to that degree of minuteness, at which it will exert a *gentle* curative influence.

§ 278. Here the question arises, as to the proper degree of reduction at which a medicine will procure certain as well as gentle relief? That is to say, how small must the dose be of each homœopathically selected medicine, in order to fulfil the requirements of a perfect cure. To determine the dose of each particular medicine for this purpose, and how to render this dose so small as to accomplish its purpose gently and rapidly at the same time, is a problem which, obviously, is neither to be solved by theoretical conjecture, nor by sophistic reasoning. Pure experiments, and accurate observation alone can solve the question; and it were folly to adduce the large doses of the old school (destitute of homœopathic bearing upon the diseased portion of the body, and affecting only the sound parts), to disprove the results of actual experience in regard to the minuteness of doses requisite to perform a homœopathic cure.

§ 279. Experience proves that *the dose of a homœopathically selected remedy cannot be reduced so far as to be inferior in strength to the natural disease, and to lose its power of extinguishing and curing at least a portion of the same, provided that this dose, immediately after having been taken, is capable of causing a slight intensification of symptoms of the similar natural disease* (slight homœopathic aggravation, §§ 157–160). This will prove to be the case in acute, chronic, and even complicated diseases, except where these depend on serious deterioration of some vital organ, or where the patient is not protected against extraneous medicinal influences.

§ 280. This incontrovertible principle, founded on experience, furnishes a standard *according to which the doses of homœopathic medicine are invariably to be reduced so far, that even after having been taken, they will merely produce an almost imperceptible homœopathic aggravation.* We should not be deterred from the use of such doses by the high degree of rarefaction that may have been reached, however incredible they may appear to the coarse material ideas of ordinary practitioners;[143] their arguments will be silenced by the verdict of infallible experience.

§ 281. In point of his disease, every patient is most susceptible to the influence of medicine, by virtue of the similitude of its effect to the disease; and there is no person, however robust, afflicted with a chronic, or so-called local disease, who would not soon perceive the desired effect in the diseased part of his body, after having taken the most minute dose of the appropriate homœopathic remedy; in other words, an *adult patient* is more easily affected by such a dose, than a *healthy* infant a day old. In view of the infallible proofs of experience, incredulity founded only upon theories, is truly insignificant and ridiculous.

§ 282. The smallest possible dose of homœopathic medicine, just strong enough to create the slightest homœopathic aggravation (because it is capable of producing symptoms which owe their power over disease to their similitude, as well as to their minuteness), will operate chiefly upon the diseased parts of the body, which have become extremely susceptible of a stimulus so similar to their own disease. The small dose will change the vital action of these parts into an artificial disease, very similar, though somewhat superior to the natural disease, and will cause the former to take the place of the latter. The organism will now contend with the artificial drug disease alone, which, according to its nature, and owing to the minuteness of the dose by which it was produced, will soon be extinguished by the vital force striving to gain its normal condition; and particularly in acute diseases, the organism will be freed from morbid processes, and restored to a healthy state.

§ 283. Proceeding quite in accordance with nature, the true physician will prescribe his well-selected homœopathic medicine in a dose so small as to be just sufficient to overcome and extinguish the disease. But as human skill and caution sometimes fail in the selection of the remedy, the smallness of the dose will certainly prevent serious injury; for the amount of disturbance arising from want of similitude and careful selection, would be so slight in consequence of so minute a dose, that the effect would soon be extinguished, or repaired by the natural vital powers, as well as by the speedy administration of an equally small dose of a more carefully chosen and similar remedy.

§ 284. The effect of a homœopathic dose is not lessened in equal proportion with the diminution of the medicinal substance contained in a dilution. A dose of eight drops of some medicinal tincture, does not produce *four times as great an effect* in the human body, as two drops would produce; but the effect would be only about twice as great as that of a two-drop dose. Hence, if one drop of a tincture is mixed with ten drops of non-medicinal liquid, and if *one drop* of this is administered, its effect will not be *ten times* greater than that of *one drop* of a mixture ten times more dilute; but the effect will be *scarcely double.* The same proportion continues to be observed, so that one drop, even of the highest dilution, may, and actually does produce a very perceptible effect.[144]

§ 285. In homœopathic practice the diminution of the dose and of effect is also conveniently accomplished by lessening the *volume* of the dose; that is, by giving a small fraction,[145] instead of a whole drop at a dose, of some medicinal dilution. This diminution of effect is readily explained by the fact that a smaller number of nerves come in contact with the medicine after the volume of its dose is divided, and although the power of the medicine is lessened, it is imparted to the whole organism.

§ 286. On the other hand, the effect of a homœopathic dose is augmented by increasing the quantity of fluid in which the medicine is dissolved preparatory to its administration, while the actual quantity of medicinal substance remains the same. In using a solution of this kind, a much greater surface supplied with sensitive nerves, susceptible of medicinal influence, is brought in contact with the medicine. Although theorists may suppose that the dilution of a dose with a greater quantity of fluid would lessen the effect, nevertheless experience in the homœopathic use of medicines, proves exactly the opposite.[146]

§ 287. When it appears desirable, before its exhibition, to augment the effect of a dose by mixing it with a greater quantity of fluid, it would make a considerable difference whether the medicinal substance of the dose is imperfectly mixed with a certain quantity of liquid, or whether it is equally and intimately[147] imparted to every particle of solvent fluid. In the latter case the solution would be far more efficacious than in the former. This will serve as a rule for the preparation of homœopathic doses, and the diminution of their medicinal effect in the treatment of very sensitive patients.[148]

§ 288. The effect of medicines in liquid form[149] penetrates and spreads through all parts of the organism with such inconceivable rapidity, from the point of contact with the sensitive nerves supplying the tissues, that this effect may, with propriety, be defined as spirit-like (dynamic or virtual).

§ 289. Every part of the body, endowed with sensitive nerves, is capable of receiving the influence of medicines, and of transmitting their power to all other parts.[150]

§ 290. Besides the stomach, the tongue and mouth are the parts most susceptible of medicinal impressions; but the lining membrane of the nose possesses this susceptibility in a high degree. Also the rectum, genitals, and all sensitive organs of our body are almost equally susceptible of medicinal effects. For this reason, parts denuded of cuticle, wounded and ulcerated surfaces, will allow the effect of medicines to penetrate quite as readily as if they had been administered by the mouth, and therefore olfaction or inhalation must be still more efficacious.

§ 291. Parts of the body deprived of their natural sense, *e. g.*, in the absence of the sense of taste or smell, the tongue, palate, and nose will impart impressions made primarily on these organs, with a considerable degree of perfection to all other organs of the body.

§ 292. Also the external surface of the body, covered by the cutis and cuticle, is capable of receiving the action particularly of liquid medicines; and the most sensitive parts of the surface are, at the same time, the most susceptible.[151]

NOTES AND EXPLANATORY REMARKS

APPENDED TO THE TEXT OF THE ORGANON.

[1] § 1. But not the habit (with which many physicians have wasted their time in search of fame), of concocting so-called systems out of certain empty vagaries and hypotheses, concerning the inner obscure nature of the process of life, or the origin of diseases; not the innumerable attempts at explaining the phenomena of diseases or their proximate cause, etc., ever hidden from their scrutiny, which were clothed in unintelligible words or as a mass of abstract phrases, intended for the astonishment of the ignorant; while suffering humanity was sighing for help. We have more than enough of such learned absurdities called *theoretical medicine*, having its own professorships, and it is high time for those who call themselves physicians, to cease deluding poor humanity by idle words, but to begin to act, that is, to help and to heal.

[2] § 6. Hence, I cannot conceive how it was possible to go to the bedside of a patient, and without carefully noting the symptoms, and being governed by them, to seek for the object of treatment in the obscure and invisible interior of the case. Neither can I understand how it was possible to pretend that the invisible, interior changes could be found and corrected by means of (unknown !) drugs, without careful consideration of symptoms, and that such could be called the only thorough and rational curative method.

Do not the sensibly discernible signs of disease represent the disease itself to the physician ? He cannot see the vital power itself, at work with immaterial forces, creating the disease; and without seeing vitality itself, he need only observe and experience its morbid effects in order to cure the disease. Why, then, must the old school seek another *prima causa morbi* in the obscure interior, while distinct sensible manifestations of disease, plainly appealing to us through symptoms, are contemptuously rejected as unworthy objects of cure. Does a cure remove anything besides these?*

[3] § 7. As a matter of course, every sensible physician will remove such causes at first; after which, the illness will generally subside of its own accord. He will remove from the sick-room flowers that may produce faintness or hysteria by their strong exhalations; he will extract irritating particles causing inflammation of the cornea; reapply to a wounded limb a bandage threatening gangrene, too tightly applied; he will avert the danger of a hæmorrhage, by exposing and tying the wounded artery; he will endeavor to expel Belladonna berries from the stomach by emetics; extract foreign substances that may have penetrated into the apertures of the body (nose, œsophagus, ears, urethra, rectum, vulva), crush a calculus, and open the occlusion of the anus of a newborn child, etc.

[4] § 8. It has ever been the habit of the old school, not knowing how else to proceed, to *single out* one of the numerous symptoms of a disease for the purpose of attacking, and, if possible, of suppressing it by medicines; *an abortive procedure* having justly excited universal contempt under the name of *symptomatic treatment*, by which nothing is gained but much is sacrificed. A single symptom is no more the disease itself, than a foot can be taken for the entire body. Such a procedure was the more objectionable, because it was the practice to treat such a single symptom only by an opposite remedy (enantiopathic and palliative), whereby, after a brief space of relief, it was made to return with greater intensity.

[5] § 8. Whenever a patient has been relieved of his disease by an adept of the true healing art, in such a manner that no sign or symptom of disease is left, and all marks of health have permanently returned, such a patient cannot, without defying common sense, be said still to have the veritable disease dwelling within him. Nevertheless, Hufeland, the leader of the old school, asserts this in the following words (v. *Homœopathie*, p. 27, L. 19): "Symptoms can be relieved by homœopathy, but the disease remains," and this assertion is made partly from grief on account of the progress of homœopathy, for the benefit of mankind, and partly because he still entertains very material notions concerning disease, which he is not yet able to consider as a dynamic

* "A physician striving to penetrate the inner conditions of the organism may err every day; the homœopathist, on the contrary, after having carefully comprehended the totality of symptoms, possesses an infallible guide, and when he has succeeded in entirely removing all the symptoms, he will certainly have cancelled the internal and obscure cause of disease."—Rau, loc. cit., p. 103.

change in the being of the organism, effected by morbidly altered vitality, nor as a modification of the state of feeling. He looks at disease as a *material thing*, which, after a cure has been effected, may still lurk in some remote corner of the body, whence it might break forth in its material presence at will, perhaps during a period of perfect health. So great is still the blindness of old-school pathologists. No wonder that therapeutics had no other object than to purge the patient.

[6] § 10. The organism is dead, and subject only to the forces of the material external world, it will decay, and again resolve itself into its chemical constituent parts.

[7] § 12. It is useless for the physician to know how the vital force brings about or creates the morbid manifestations of the organism, and therefore it will ever remain obscure; only that which it was necessary for him to know concerning disease, and sufficient for the purpose of cure, has been revealed to his senses.

[8] § 17. A prophetic dream, a superstition, or the solemn prophecy that death would assuredly occur on a certain day, or at a certain hour, has not infrequently caused the appearance of every sign of approaching and increasing fatal disease, or of death itself at the designated time; a result which would have been impossible, without the occurrence of an internal change corresponding with the externally visible condition. In the same way, all morbid signs of approaching death were frequently dispelled, and health suddenly restored by an artful deception, or convincing denial. This would have been equally impossible without the effect of these moral remedies, by means of which the death-bringing internal and external morbid changes were removed.

[9] § 17. And thus, the goodness of Providence was made known to us by revealing that part of diseases to the physician, which it was his duty to remove, in order to end them, and to reëstablish health. We would never have become conscious of Divine goodness and wisdom in regard to diseases if, as has been pretended by the old school (which claims the power of divining the inner nature of things), that curable part of them had been hidden from our senses by mysterious darkness, and secluded in the interior of the body, making it impossible for man to recognize the evil distinctly, and equally impossible to cure it.

[10] § 22. The only other method besides the two above named, of prescribing medicines (*the allopathic method*), having symptoms of no

direct specific (pathical) relation to the diseased condition; and which are neither similar nor opposed, but heterogeneous to the symptoms of the disease; that method, as I have shown above in the *Introduction* (Review of "Physic," etc.), is merely an imperfect and pernicious imitation of the hurtful endeavors of the unreasoning, instinctive vital force, disturbed by hurtful influences, and trying to regain its equilibrium at all hazards, by inciting and maintaining a diseased condition in the organism. It is consequently an imitation of the crude vital force, created in and together with our organism, in order to preserve the perfect harmony of life. But this same vital force, if disturbed during disease, is to be again restored to the harmony of health by the (homœopathic) interference of the intelligent physician. It is not meant that it should cure itself, and its unsuccessful attempts are quite unworthy of imitation; because all changes of feeling produced by the disturbed vital force in the organism, actually constitute the disease itself. Still, it would be as improper to leave this inappropriate practice of the old school of medicine unnoticed, as it would be to omit in the history of man those instances of oppression, from which the human race has suffered for thousands of years under despotic and unreasonable governments.

[11] § 25. I do not mean the experience boasted of by ordinary practitioners of the old school, who have wantonly applied a lot of complex recipes in numerous diseases never properly investigated, but dogmatically considered as already well defined by pathology, and to contain an imaginary morbific matter, or some other hypothetical internal abnormity. They invariably perceive something, without knowing what it is, and experience results which no man can single out from among the manifold forces acting upon the unknown object; no useful knowledge could be gained from such results. Fifty years of such experience is equal to gazing for fifty years into a kaleidoscope, filled with many colored unknown things, and constantly made to revolve—a thousand changeable forms, but no clue to them!

[12] § 26. In this manner physical affections as well as moral evils are cured. How does Jupiter, shining brightly in the morning dawn, vanish from the optic nerve of the beholder? By a stronger potency, the brightness of approaching day, similar in its action upon the optic nerve. By what are the olfactory nerves effectually soothed when they have been offended by offensive odors? By snuff, which is similar but stronger in its action upon the sense of smell. Neither music, nor sweetmeats, which bear a relation to the nerves of other senses, will cure that loathing of odors. How cunningly the soldier knows how to guard the ears of the bystanders, from the whimpering tones of one condemned to run the gauntlet—by the shrill squeaking fife, accom-

panied by the noisy drum. How does a soldier counteract fear created in his army, by the distant thunder of the enemies' guns? By the deep, droning sound of the great drum. Neither case would have been remedied by the distribution of glittering accoutrements, nor by a reprimanding order issued to the regiment. In the same manner, grief and sorrow are extinguished in the mind by more intense, real, or fictitious affliction of another person. The evil consequences of overjoy are relieved by coffee, which produces a feeling of excessive joyfulness. Nations like the Germans, degraded for centuries by listless apathy and abject submissiveness, were to be trodden in the dust by the Conqueror from the West, until oppression became intolerable. Thus their feelings of self-degradation were overcome and neutralized, they became conscious of their dignity as human beings once more, and again could lift their heads as German men.

[13] § 29. Artificial morbific potencies which we call medicines, though stronger than natural diseases, are nevertheless more easily overcome by the vital force, owing to the brief period of action of these medicines; while the diseases being of chronic and of lifelong duration (psora, syphilis, sycosis), are never conquered and extinguished by the vital power alone, until the physician reinforces it by means of a similar, and, therefore, morbific potency (homœopathic drug). This, when taken internally (or by olfaction) is forced, as it were, upon the instinctive vital power, and substituted in the place of the hitherto dominant natural disease; thereupon the vital power merely remains affected by the drug, but only for a short time; because the effect of the drug (the space of time required by the drug-disease to run its course), does not continue long. Diseases protracted for years, which have been cured by an eruption of small-pox and of measles (both having a duration of several weeks), are processes of a similar nature.

[14] § 31. When I designate a disease as a modification or *discordancy* of the state of health of the human body, I am far from presuming to attempt metaphysical explanation of the inner nature of diseases in general, or of any disease in particular. Such are only intended to indicate what diseases evidently *are not* and *cannot* be, viz., not mechanical or chemical changes of the material body; nor are they dependent on material morbific matter, but merely spiritual dynamic disturbances of life.

[15] § 33. A notable instance of this kind is, that previous to the year 1801, the smooth form of scarlatina of Sydenham, prevailed from time to time as an epidemic among children, invariably attacking those who had not suffered from it during a previous epidemic: while, during an epidemic like the one I witnessed at Königslutter, *all* children re-

mained unaffected by this highly contagious disease, whenever they had taken in good season, a very small dose of Belladonna. If drugs can guard against infection from an epidemic disease, they must necessarily possess a superior power of modifying our vital force.

[16] § 36. *Mémoires et Observationes, in the Description de l'Egypte*, Tom. I.

[17] § 38. Obs., lib. I, 8.

[18] § 38. In *Hufeland's Journal*, XV, ii.

[19] § 38. Chevalier, in *Hufeland's Neuesten Annalen der französichen Heilkunde* (*Newest Annals of French Medicine*).

[20] § 38. *Mania phthisi superveniens eam cum omnibus suis phænomenis auffert, verum mox redit phthisis et occidit, abeunte mania. Reil. Memorab. Fasc.*, III, v, p. 171.

[21] § 38. In *Edin. Med. Comment.*, Part I, 1.

[22] § 38. John Hunter on *Venereal Diseases*, p. 5.

[23] § 38. Rainay, in *Med. Comment. of Edinb.*, III, p. 480.

[24] § 38. It was also very correctly described by Withering and Plenciz, but it is very different from purple rash (or *Roodvonk*), which was erroneously called scarlet fever. Only during the last year, both diseases, though originally very different, have become approximated in regard to their symptoms.

[25] § 38. Jenner, in *Medicinische Annalen*, 1800, August, p. 747.

[26] § 38. In *Hufeland's Journal der Practischen Arzneikunde*, XX, iii, p. 50.

[27] § 38. Loc. cit.

[28] § 39. *Obs, Phys. Med.*, Lib. 2, obs. 30.

[29] § 40. After exact experiments and cures of this kind of complicated diseases, I have arrived at the conviction that the two diseases are not blended together, but that in such cases, they merely exist side by side in the organism, each one dwelling in the parts for which it has an affinity; since their perfect cure is effected by a well-timed al-

ternation of the best mercurial preparation, with remedies for the cure of the itch; each to be administered in appropriate dose and preparation.

[30] § 40. *Transactions of a Society for the improvement of Medical and Chirurgical Knowledge*, II.

[31] § 40. In *Med. Comment. of Edin.*, III, p. 480.

[32] § 40. In *Med. and Phys. Journ.*, 1805.

[33] § 40. *Opera*, II, p. i, cap. 10.

[34] § 40. In *Hufeland's Journal*, XVII.

[35] § 41. Besides the morbific symptoms which, by virtue of their similitude, possess the power of curing homœopathically the venereal disease, quicksilver, in its mode of action, evinces many others dissimilar to syphilis which, in the frequent cases of complication with psora, are productive of new evils, and of great destruction in the body.

[36] § 45. See above, footnote to § 26.

[37] § 45. In the same manner as the image of a candle-flame is speedily overpowered (überstimmt) and erased from the optic nerve, by a stronger sunbeam falling upon the eye.

[38] § 46. *Traité de l'inoculation*, p. 189.

[39] § 46. *Heilkunde für Mütter*, p. 384.

[40] § 46. *Interpres Clinicus*, p. 293.

[41] § 46. *Neue Heilart der Kinderpocken*, Ulm, 1769, p. 68, and *Specim. obs.*, No. 18.

[42] § 46. Loc. cit.

[43] § 46. *Nov. act. Nat. cur.*, vol. I, obs. 22.

[44] § 46. *Nachricht von dem Kranken-Institut zu Erlangen*, 1783.

[45] § 46. Robert Willan on *Vaccination*.

[46] § 46. Particularly Clavier, Hurel, and Desormeaux, in the *Bul-*

letin des Soc. Médicales, publié par les Mémbres du Comité Central de la Soc. de Médecine du Département de l'Eure, 1808; also in the *Journal de Médecine Continué*, vol. xv, p. 206.

[47] § 46. Balhorn, in *Hufeland's Journal*, X, ii.

[48] § 46. Stevenson in *Duncan's Annals of Medicine*, Lustr. II, vol. i, dis. 3, No. 9.

[49] § 46. In *Hufeland's Journ. der pr. Arzneik.* XXIII.

[50] § 46. *On Venereal Disease*, p. 4.

[51] § 46. *Elemens de Médec. prat. de M. Cullen, Traduits*, P. II, 1, 3, ch. 7.

[52] § 46. Or that symptom, at least, was removed.

[53] § 46. In *Hufeland's Journal*, XX, iii, p. 50.

[54] § 46. *Rau, über d. Werth des Homœop. Heilverfahrens.* Heidelb., 1824, p. 85.

[55] § 50. And the contagious humor of another contagious disease, carried along as a secondary ingredient of vaccine matter.

[56] § 50. Namely, small-pox and measles.

[57] § 52. See above, in the Introduction: *Review of Physic*, etc., and my book, *Allopathie, ein Wort der Warnung für Kranke jeder Art.* (*Allopathy, a Word of Warning for Sufferers of all Kinds*). Leipzig, by Baumgärtner.

[58] § 55. *Review of Physic*, etc.

[59] § 56. The attempt is made by some to create a fourth mode of applying medicines in diseases, by means of *isopathy*, as it is called; that is, to cure an equal disease by an equal miasm. But supposing this were possible—and it would deserve the name of a valuable discovery—the cure in that case could only be accomplished by opposing a *similimum* to a *similimum*, since isopathy administers only a highly potentiated, and, as it were, altered miasm to a patient.

[60] § 58. Little as physicians have been in the habit of observing, the aggravations following such palliatives could not have escaped their

attention. A good example of this kind may be found in J. H. Schulze, *Diss. qua corporis humani momentanearum alterationum specimina quædam expenduntur, Halæ*, 1741, § 28. Something of a similar nature is stated by Willis, *Pharm. rat.*, sect. 7, cap. I, p. 298: "Opiata dolores atrocissimos plerumque sedant atque indolentiam—procurant, eamque—aliquamdiu et pro stato quodam tempore continuant, quo spatio elapso, dolores mox recrudescunt et brevi ad solitam ferociam augentur." And further on, p. 295: "Exactis opii viribus illico redeunt tormina, nec atrocitatem suam remittunt, nisi dum ab eodem pharmaco rursus incantantur." J. Hunter says (*On Venereal Disease*, p. 13), that wine increases the activity of the weak, without imparting true strength to them, and that the strength afterwards declines in proportion to the previous stimulation, whereby no advantage is gained, but that the strength is mostly wasted.

[61] § 59. See Introduction, towards the end.

[62] § 59. See Hufeland's pamphlet, *Die Homœopathie*, p. 20.

[63] § 67. Only in cases of extreme urgency, where danger and imminent death do not afford sufficient time for the action of a homœopathic remedy, leaving it scarcely an hour, a quarter of an hour, or even minutes, to take effect, it is necessary to make use of palliatives. For instance, in sudden attacks befalling previously healthy persons, such as asphyxia, and apparent death from lightning, suffocation, freezing, drowning, etc., it would be appropriate and to the purpose to stimulate at first the susceptibility and sensibility (physical life), by mild electric shocks, injections of strong coffee, by stimulating the olfactories, by applying gradual warmth, etc. As soon as life is again manifested, the action of vital organs resumes its previous healthy course, because, in this instance, no disease,* but only a suspension or suppression of vital force, which was in itself healthy, was to be removed. Various antidotes to sudden cases of poisoning are here in place, such as alkalies for mineral acids, liver of sulphur for metallic poisons, coffee, camphor (and Ipecacuanha) for opium poisoning, etc. A homœopathic medicine is not necessarily selected improperly for a disease, if a few drug-symptoms should happen to bear only an antipathic relation to some of its intermediate and minor symptoms, as

* Nevertheless the new sect appeals to this remark, in order to find such exceptions to the rule everywhere in diseases, by way of pretext for the application of their allopathic palliatives and other pernicious devices, only for the sake of avoiding the trouble of finding the right homœopathic remedy for every case of disease; or, as one might say, to avoid the trouble of being homœopathic physicians, as which, however, they wish to appear; but their deeds are in conformity with their aspirations; they are insignificant.

long as the other, stronger, particularly prominent (characteristic) symptoms of the disease are properly covered, that is, overcome and extinguished (homœopathically) by the symptom-similitude of the same remedy. The few contrary symptoms will then vanish spontaneously, after the time of action of the medicine has passed, and the cure will not be retarded in the least.

[64] § 69. Permanent neutralization of conflicting or antagonistic sensations, never occurs in the living body as it does in the chemical laboratory, with substances of opposite properties, *e. g.*, where sulphuric acid and potassa unite to form a neutral salt, an entirely different substance, neither acid nor alkaline, and which cannot even be decomposed by lime. A blending or intimate reunion of this kind, resulting in something permanently neutral and indifferent, cannot be brought about, as above stated, by dynamic impressions of opposite nature in our organs of sensation. Only an apparent neutralization, or mutual obliteration takes place in such a case, but opposite sensations do not cancel each other permanently. The tears of a sorrowful person are arrested but for a short time by a merry spectacle, but he will soon forget the ludicrous impression, and his tears will flow more copiously afterwards.

[65] § 69. Unmistakable as this is, it has nevertheless been misunderstood, and the objection raised, "that the palliative in its after-effect being the similar of the present disease, would probably effect a cure as well as a homœopathic medicine would do in its primary effect." But it was overlooked that the after-effect is not the product of the medicine, but always of the counteracting vital force of the organism ; and, hence this after-effect, produced by the vital force upon the application of a palliative, is only a condition resembling the disease-symptom left unextinguished by the palliative ; and consequently *aggravated* by the counteraction of the vital force against the palliative.

[66] § 69. Like the effect which might be produced by the sudden ignition of alcohol in a dark dungeon, where the prisoner can discern near objects but imperfectly, the flame would at first exhibit everything to the sufferer in a comforting light ; but the brighter the flame had been, so much the darker would be the night surrounding the prisoner, obscuring objects more deeply than before.

[67] § 73. The homœopathic physician, unbiassed by the prejudices of the common school (which had affixed certain names to such fevers, besides which great nature was expected to produce no others, in order that their treatment, framed after a certain pattern, need not be inter-

fered with), does not recognize appellations like those of dungeon-fever, bilious fever, typhus fever, putrid fever, nervous and mucous fever, but treats each one according to its peculiarities.

[68] § 73. Subsequent to the year 1801, a kind of purple-rash (roodvonk), introduced from western countries, was mistaken by physicians for scarlet fever, although the one was distinguished from the other by very different signs, the former being prevented and cured by Aconite, the latter by Belladonna, and while the former occurred sporadically, the latter was always an epidemic. In later years, both have at times appeared united in a peculiar form of eruptive fever, to which neither of the above remedies longer correspond singly.

[69] § 74. When the patient finally succumbs, the physician who has treated him, usually exhibits, during a post-mortem examination, these organic changes to the mourning relatives, cunningly representing the consequences of his want of skill, as the original and incurable evil (cf. my book, *Allopathy, a Word of Warning to Patients of all Kinds*, Leips., by Baumgärtner). Illustrated works on morbid anatomy, calling to mind deceptive reminiscences, contain the product of such poor treatment.

[70] § 79. I have devoted twelve years to the discovery of the source of these exceedingly numerous chronic maladies, to the investigation and realization of the great truth hitherto unknown to our predecessors and contemporaries, and, at the same time, to the discovery of the principal (antipsoric) remedies, which in their various manifestations and forms, would in most instances prove to be of superior strength in combating this many-headed monster. My experiences concerning this matter, have been given in the book entitled, *The Chronic Diseases* (2 parts, Dresden: Arnold, 1828, 1830). Before I had succeeded in gaining a clear view of the subject, I could only recommend that all chronic diseases should be treated as other distinct cases, by means of medicinal substances, according to their effect, as derived from the provings hitherto made upon healthy persons. Hence, my pupils treated each case of chronic disease like others of a peculiar kind ; and they often succeeded so far in curing it, that suffering humanity rejoiced in the progress of the fertile resources of the new healing art. How much greater should be the cause for contentment, now that the desired object is so near its consummation, since the newly discovered, and more highly specific homœopathic remedies (properly called antipsorics) for chronic diseases, originated by psora, have been made known, together with their methods of preparation and application in disease. But of their number the true physician selects for healing purposes, those of which the drug-symptoms are most similar

to the chronic disease they are intended to cure, thereby insuring more essential services, and almost invariable success from (antipsoric) medicines more adapted to this miasm.

[71] § 81. Some of these causes which so modify the development of psora as to produce chronic evils, obviously depend in part on climate and natural peculiarities of habitations, and partly on improper moral and physical education of the young; on the neglect, distortion, or over-training of both mind and body; on the abuse of bodily and mental functions in vocations and other conditions of life; of dietetic habits, human passions, customs, and fashions of various kinds.

[72] § 81. Pathology has given rise to many misapplied and ambiguous names, each of which is applied to very different morbid conditions, often having but a single symptom in common, such as *ague, jaundice, dropsy, consumption, leucorrhœa, hæmorrhoids, rheumatism, apoplexy, convulsions, hysteria, hypochondriasis, melancholy, mania, croup, paralysis, etc.*, which are described as fixed, unvarying diseases, and treated by name according to an undeviating routine. Is it justifiable to base medicinal treatment on a mere name? Or, if it is otherwise, why is the same kind of treatment always predetermined by identical names? "Nihil sane in artem medicam pestiferum magis unquam irrepsit malum, quam generalia quædam nomina morbis imponere, iisque aptare velle generalem quandam medicinam," says Huxham, whose conscientiousness deserves as much respect as his keen insight (*Op. Phys. Med.*, tom. I.). In a similar manner Fritze complains (*Annalen*, I, p. 80), "that essentially different diseases are designated by one name." Those general diseases even, which are undoubtedly propagated *in each particular epidemic*, by a peculiar kind of contagious matter of unknown nature, have names assigned to them by the old school of medicine, as if they always returned in the same well-known and established form, such as *hospital, dungeon, camp, putrid, bilious, nervous, mucous fevers;* notwithstanding that each epidemic of these wandering fevers, may always be distinguished as a different and *new* disease, never known before in precisely the same form, differing from others in its course, as well as in many of its most prominent symptoms, and in its general features as exhibited for the time being. Each one is so unlike all other preceding epidemics, whatever their names, that it would be a violation of logical accuracy, if we were to attach one of those pathological terms to these heterogeneous disorders, and then treat them according to this misapplied name. This was already observed by the honest Sydenham, who insists (Oper., cap. 2, *de Morb. Epid.*, p. 43), that no epidemic disease should be considered as having occurred before, or treated according to a method applied on a previous occasion, since all of them, regardless of the number of successive

epidemics, were different from each other: "Animum admiratione percellit, quam discolor et sui plane dissimilis morborum epidemicorum facies; quæ tam aperta horum morborum diversitas tum propriis ac sibi peculiaribus symptomatis tum etiam medendi ratione, quam hi ab illis disparem sibi vindicant, satis illucescit. Ex quibus constat, morbos epidemicos, utut externa quatantenus specie et symptomatis aliquot utrisque pariter convenire paullo incautioribus videantur, re tamen ipsa, si bene adverteris animum, alienæ esse admodum indolis et distare ut æra lupinis."

From all this it becomes evident that these useless and inapplicable names of diseases should not be permitted to control the method of cure employed by a true physician, who knows that diseases are never to be discerned or cured according to the similarity of names which refer to single symptoms, but in conformity with the totality of every symptom of the particular condition peculiar to each patient, whose suffering must be accurately investigated. but never hypothetically assumed.

If, however, names of diseases are occasionally needed for the sake of brevity, while speaking of a patient in popular language, they should be used only as collective names; thus, for instance, we might say the patient has *a kind of* St. Vitus's dance, *a kind of* dropsy, *a kind of* nervous fever, *a kind of* ague; but (in order to avoid all this delusive nomenclature) we should never say he has *the* St. Vitus's dance, *the* nervous fever, *the* dropsy, *the* ague; because fixed and unvarying diseases with these names, actually have no existence.

[73] § 82. The plan laid down in the following paragraphs, concerning the investigation of symptoms, only partially refers to acute diseases.

[74] § 84. Every interruption disturbs the course of thought of the narrator, who will subsequently be unable to recall his ideas precisely in that form in which he would have expressed them at the outset.

[75] § 87. The physician should not put his question thus, for example: "Did you not observe this or that circumstance?" He should not make any suggestions, leading to a deceptive answer and statement.

[76] § 88. The physician should ask, for example: "What is the condition of your bowels? How does the urine pass? What have you to say about your sleep in the daytime, as well as at night? What is your frame of mind, your moods, or your power of memory? How is it with regard to thirst? What sort of taste do you experience in your mouth? What food or drink do you relish most? What is most

distasteful to you? Has your food or drink its natural full taste, or a strange and different one? How do you feel after eating or drinking? Have you anything to remark about your head, limbs, or abdomen?"

[77] § 89. For example, questions should be put as follows: "How often do you have an evacuation from the bowels, and what is the precise character of the discharge? Was the whitish discharge mucus, or fecal matter? Were there any pains during the evacuation or not? What kind of pains, and where? What did the patient vomit up? Is the disagreeable taste in the mouth foul, bitter, sour, or otherwise? Do you experience it before, after, or during eating or drinking? At what time of the day is it most perceptible? Of what taste are the eructations? Does the urine become turbid on standing in the vessel, or is it turbid while passing? Of what color is the water just after passing it? What is the color of the sediment? How do you act, or what do you feel while sleeping? Does he whimper, groan, talk, or cry out in his sleep? Does he start in sleep? Does the patient snore with the in- or expiration? Does he lie only on his back, or on which side? Does he cover himself snugly, or does he not allow himself to be covered? Does he awake easily, or does he sleep too soundly? How does he feel directly after awaking from sleep? How often do you experience this or that complaint, and upon what occasions does it come? While sitting, lying, standing, or during exercise? During an empty stomach, or at least in the morning, or only at night, or only after a meal, or at what other times? When did the rigor take place? Was it merely a feeling of chilliness, or was the patient cold at the time? In which parts? Or was he even hot to the touch during the feeling of chilliness? Was it only a feeling of coldness without shuddering? Was he hot without being red in the face? Which parts felt cold to the touch? Or did he complain of heat, without actually feeling cold to the touch? What was the duration of the chill and of the heat? When did thirst set in? During the chill? During the heat? Before it or after it? How severe was the thirst, and for what? When does the perspiration set in, in the beginning or at the end of the heat? Or how many hours after the heat? While sleeping, or waking? How profuse was the perspiration? Was it hot, or cold? On which parts? Of what odor? What does the patient complain of before, or during the chill? Of what, during the heat? Of what, afterwards? Of what, during or after the perspiration?" etc.

[78] § 90. He should note, for instance, how the patient behaved during the visit, whether morose, quarrelsome, hasty, inclined to weep, anxious, despairing or sorrowful, or confident and calm, etc.; note down if he was somnolent, or without recollection; if he spoke hoarsely, in a whisper, or if his language was improper or otherwise; note the

complexion of the face, and the color of the eyes and skin in general; the vivacity and force of features and eyes; the condition of the tongue, breath, and the odor from the mouth, and also the hearing; how much the pupils were dilated or contracted; how rapidly or how much they are inclined to change in darkness and in light; note the state of the pulse, of the abdomen, how moist or how hot it is; how cold or dry the skin is in general, or in particular parts; notice the patient's position, if lying with his mouth open partially or widely, if his arms are thrown above his head, if he lies on his back or otherwise; with what degree of effort he raises himself up, and every other striking observation regarding the patient, should be noted by the physician.

[79] § 93. Circumstances, the disclosure of which reflects disgrace upon the patient, and which are not readily or willingly mentioned by him or his attendants, must be traced out by the physician through skilfully constructed questions or private inquiries. The following may be enumerated in this class: Poisoning or attempted suicide; masturbation; sexual excesses of ordinary or unnatural kind; abuse of wine, liquors, punch, and other heating beverages, including coffee; over-eating in general, or of particularly hurtful food; infection with venereal disease, or the itch; unrequited love; jealousy; domestic discord; mortification; grief in consequence of family misfortunes; maltreatment; suppressed feeling of revenge; humiliation; pecuniary losses; superstitious fear; want; malformation of sexual organs; hernia; prolapsus, etc.

[80] § 94. In chronic diseases of the female sex, particular attention should be paid to pregnancy, sterility, inclination to sexual intercourse, childbirth, abortions, suckling, and the condition of the menstrual discharge. Especially in regard to the latter, the inquiry should not be neglected, whether it returns too early or is delayed beyond the regular time; how many days it lasts, continuously or interruptedly; its quantity should be ascertained, as well as its color; whether preceded or followed by leucorrhœa (whites); particular notice should be taken of the accompanying bodily and mental complaints, sensations and pains before, during, and after the appearance of the menstrual discharge. Is it combined with leucorrhœa, and of what kind? With what sensations? In what quantity, under which conditions, and on what occasions does it appear?

[81] § 96. Purely fictitious accounts of morbid attacks and complaints, will scarcely be met with in the case of even the most incorrigible hypochondriacs; this is plainly proved by comparing their accounts of complaints given at different times, while the physician has administered nothing, or merely non-medicinal things. It is only

necessary to make certain deductions from their exaggerations, or at least the force of their expressions should be accredited to their overwrought feelings; in this respect an exaggerated statement of their complaints should be set down by itself in the list of the rest of significant symptoms, composing the picture of the disease. The case is different with maniacs, and those who viciously simulate disease.

[82] § 102. If the physician had been able to select in the first cases the appropriate remedy, nearly approaching a homœopathic specific, the subsequent cases will either confirm the appropriateness of the chosen remedy, or point out a still more suitable, or the most suitable homœopathic remedy.

[83] § 104. Physicians of the old school make very light of the matter. With them a careful inquiry into all the circumstances of the patient was unheard of. The physician would even interrupt patients in the narration of their complaints, that he might be undisturbed in hastily writing off a recipe, composed of numerous ingredients, of which the real effects were unknown to him. No allopathic physician then demanded information concerning every particular circumstance of the patient, *and still less would he write down anything* concerning him. On revisiting the patient after several days, he remembered little or nothing of what he had heard (having seen so many different patients in the meantime); what he had heard with one ear, escaped from the other. Nor would he ask more than a few general questions during subsequent visits; he would seem to feel the pulse at the wrist, look at the tongue, prescribe another recipe at the same moment, also without good reason, or order the former prescription to be continued (frequently throughout the day, in considerable doses), and then depart most gracefully to visit the fiftieth or sixtieth patient, in a single forenoon, in order to go through with the same senseless routine. In this way people, calling themselves physicians, and rational physicians at that, made a business of a profession, actually requiring more earnest thought than any other in the conscientious and careful investigation of the condition of each patient, to serve as a basis for the special mode of treatment. The result was almost invariably unfavorable; nevertheless, patients were obliged to resort to these physicians, partly for want of better ones, and partly from courtesy.

[84] § 108. During the past twenty-five hundred years, as far as I know, not a single physician, with the exception of the great and immortal Albrecht von Haller, has hit upon this method of proving (testing) drugs with reference to their pure and peculiar effects, by altering the sensorial condition of man, which furnishes the most natural and indispensable means of discovering what morbid conditions each

drug is capable of curing. Excepting myself, Haller was the only one who recognized this necessity (cf. the preface to the *Pharmacopœia Helvet.*, Basil, 1771, fol., p. 12): "Nempe primum in corpore *sano* medela tentanda est, *sine peregrina ulla miscela;* odoreque et sapore ejus exploratis, exigua illius dosis ingerenda et ad omnes, quæ inde contingunt, affectiones, quis pulsus, qui calor, quæ respiratio, quænam excretiones, attendendum. Inde ad ductum phænomenorum, in sano obviorum, transeas ad experimenta in corpore ægroto, etc." But no physician has ever obeyed these invaluable hints.

[85] § 106. Besides pure homœopathy, another true and more perfect way of healing dynamic (*i. e.*, all non-surgical) diseases cannot exist, as it is impossible to draw more than one straight line between two given points. How little must he who imagines there are still other kinds of diseases to be cured, besides those amenable to homœopathy, have penetrated into its depth, or how insufficiently must he have practiced it; how few correctly planned homœopathic cures must he have seen or read of, and, on the other hand, how imperfectly must he have weighed in his mind the absence of any foundation in every allopathic mode of procedure, or have acquired information concerning their poor, nay, horrible results; who, with shallow indifference, considers the merits of the only true healing art as equal to those pernicious modes of treatment, or who even pretends that they are the sisters of homœopathy, and indispensable to it. My true and conscientious followers may refute such notions by their almost unerring fortunate cures.

[86] § 106. I have deposited the fruits of these researches in the degree of perfection they had attained up to that time in *Fragmenta de viribus medicamentorum positivis, sive in sano corp. num. observatis*, Part I, II, Leipsiæ, 8, 1805, apud J. A. Barth; the riper ones in the pure *Materia Medica*, Part I, third ed., Part II, third ed., 1833; Part III, second ed., 1825; Part IV, second ed., 1825; Part V, second ed., 1826; Part VI, second ed., 1827; and in the second, third, and fourth parts of the *Chronic Diseases*, 1828, 1830. Dresden, by Arnold.

[87] § 110. Compare what I have said regarding this matter in the *Illustration of the Sources of the Common Materia Medica*, preceding the third part of my *Pure Materia Medica.*

[88] § 117. Some persons are made to faint away by the odor of roses, and may be affected by a variety of morbid and sometimes dangerous conditions after partaking of limpets, craw-fish, or of the spawn of the barb, or from touching the leaves of some kind of sumach, etc.

[89] § 117. In this manner the Princess Maria Porphyrogeneta re-

lieved her brother, the Emperor Alexius, suffering from fainting attacks, by sprinkling him with rose-water (τὸ τῶν ῥόδων στάλαγμα) in the presence of his aunt Eudoxia (*Hist. Byz. Alexias*, lib. 15, p. 503, ed. Posser), and Horstius (Oper., III, p. 59) found rose-vinegar very efficacious in cases of fainting.

[90] § 118. This was also recognized by the distinguished von Haller, when he says (preface to his *Hist. Stirp Helv.*): "Latet immensa virium diversitas in iis ipsis plantis, quarum facies externas dudum novimus, animas quasi et quodcunque cælestius habent, nondum perspeximus."

[91] § 119. Whoever is acquainted with the peculiar effect of each particular substance upon the state of human feelings, and whoever knows how to appreciate it, will readily comprehend that in regard to their medicinal qualities there can be among these remedies none of equivalent value, or that could be *substituted* for each other. Only he who is *unacquainted* with the pure and positive effects of the different drugs, can be guilty of the folly of trying to persuade us that one could serve instead of the other, or that one might be as useful as the other in the same disease. In this way unreasonable children confound essentially different things, because they can hardly distinguish them according to their exterior, and least of all, according to their value, their true significance, and their extremely diversified properties.

[92] § 119. If this is the truth, as it certainly is, no physician, unwilling to be regarded as unreasonable, or to disturb his clear conscience, the only mark of man's true dignity, will henceforth apply a medicine in the treatment of diseases, unless he is fully and exactly informed of its true significance, *i. e.*, the virtual effect of which, upon the condition of healthy persons, he has explored so thoroughly, that he is perfectly sure of its ability to produce a very similar morbid condition, one more similar than that of every other drug, equally well known to him, to the disease to be cured; for as has been shown above, neither man nor great nature herself can heal perfectly, rapidly, and permanently but by means of a homœopathic remedy. No real physician can henceforth forego such experiments, in order to obtain the most necessary and only knowledge of drugs for healing purposes—this knowledge hitherto neglected by physicians of all past ages. Posterity will scarcely believe that in all past centuries up to the present day, physicians were content to treat diseases by blindly prescribing medicines of unknown significance, and *unproved* with regard to their highly important, diversified, and pure dynamic effects upon the human condition; nay, to administer several of these unknown and widely different powers compounded in one recipe, and to leave chance to direct the result upon the patient. This is the way in which a maniac would enter the studio of an artist,

seizing handfuls of very different and unfamiliar implements, wherewith to complete, as he imagines, the works of art he sees before him. That these will be injured and irreparably ruined by him, it is unnecessary for me to add.

[93] § 125. New green peas, beans, and perhaps carrots are admissible as being probably the least medicinal among green vegetables.

[94] § 125. The prover should either be unaccustomed to undiluted wine, spirits, coffee or tea, or should for some time previously have given up the use of these stimulating, and otherwise medicinally hurtful beverages.

[95] § 139. Whoever makes such experiments known to the medical profession, becomes responsible for the reliability of the proving person, and the statements of the latter, and justly so, since the welfare of suffering humanity is involved.

[96] § 141. By making his own person the subject of experiments, the physician will derive many other invaluable advantages. First of all, the great truth will appear to the physician in the light of an incontrovertible fact that the medicinal quality of all drugs, the basis of their healing power, lies in the changes of sensorial condition perceived by himself, and in the morbid conditions personally observed as the result of drugs proved upon himself. Furthermore, the necessity of bestowing such close attention upon the remarkable phenomena appearing in his own person, will partly lead him to comprehend the significance of his own feelings, and of his own habits of thought and temperament (the foundation of all true wisdom, γνῶθι σεαυτόν), and partly it will educate him to be an observer, an attribute which no physician should lack. All our observations made upon others fail to exercise the attraction we feel while experimenting upon ourselves. The observer of others must necessarily always fear that the prover of a drug may not have felt everything as distinctly as he says, or that he may not have stated his feelings in the appropriate expression. He is ever in doubt lest he may have been partially deceived. This almost unavoidable obstacle to the recognition of the truth in eliciting information about disease-symptoms artificially originated by drugs upon others, is naturally precluded from the experiments made upon one's own person. A self-prover knows with certainty what he has felt, and every experiment of the kind made upon himself stimulates him to explore the powers of numerous other drugs. In this manner he will grow more and more expert in the art of observing, so indispensable to a physician as long as he continues to make himself the infallible and undeceptive subject of his observations; he will perceive with all the more ardor, because these experiments upon himself, without deceiving him, promise to

teach him the true value and significance of many yet missing agents necessary for healing purposes. No fear should be entertained that such slight ailments, called forth by taking drugs that are to be proved, would ever be detrimental to the health of the prover. Experience teaches, on the contrary, that the organism of the prover, by repeated attacks upon the healthy condition, will become all the more accustomed to repel everything of an injurious character attacking the body from without, as well as all kinds of artificial and natural morbific influences, and that the organism will become inured to everything of a deleterious nature by means of these moderate experiments with drugs.

[97] § 142. Symptoms observed, either in past stages of the disease or not at all, and which, therefore, must have been new symptoms peculiar to the drug.

[98] § 143. In modern times, distant and unknown persons have been employed and paid for proving drugs, and their reports have been printed. But this most important business, destined to lay the foundation for the only true healing art, and demanding the most positive moral certainty in its results, seems to become ambiguous and unreliable by such practice, and to lose all its value.

[99] § 145. At first I was the only one who made the proving of medicinal powers the most important of all his duties. Since that time I have been assisted in this by a number of young men, who have made experiments upon themselves, and whose observations I have carefully reviewed. But what grand curative results will be obtained within the whole circumference of the endless realm of diseases, as soon as a greater number of *accurate and reliable* observers shall have enriched this only genuine science of Materia Medica by meritorious *experiments upon themselves!* The calling of the physician will then approach the infallibility of mathematical sciences.

[100] § 145. Compare note 86, § 109.

[101] § 149. But this often very laborious search and selection of a homœopathic remedy adapted in every respect to the morbid condition in hand, is a business demanding the study of the original sources, and much careful circumspection, as well as serious reflection, notwithstanding the existence of many praiseworthy books intended to facilitate the burdens of an office, which finds its highest reward alone in the consciousness of having faithfully fulfilled a duty. How can this laborious, careful occupation, which alone furnishes the possibility of accomplishing the best cures of diseases, be expected to suit the convenience of the members of a new mongrel sect, who boast with the honorable title of

homœopathist, and who, for the sake of appearance, make prescriptions in the form and character of homœopathic medicines, merely snatched up (*quidquid in buccam venit*) at haphazard, and who, if the inaccurately chosen remedy does not bring immediate relief, do not throw the blame upon their inexcusable indolence and carelessness in transacting the most important and serious affairs of mankind, but who saddle the fault upon homœopathy, accusing it of great imperfections (perhaps because it does not supply them with the proper homœopathic remedy for every morbid condition without any trouble on their part, after the manner of certain fabulous pigeons that flew, ready roasted, into an open mouth?). But like smart people, they do not allow their want of success, occasioned by their scarcely half-homœopathic remedies, to trouble them; they resort at once to their more familiar allopathic hobbies, among which a dozen or so of leeches, applied to the painful part, or a little innocent bloodletting of about eight ounces, etc., serves to make a very favorable appearance; and, if the patient recovers in spite of all this, they praise their bloodletting, leeches, etc., saying that without these the patient could not have been saved; and they try to have it distinctly understood that these operations, derived, without much deliberation, from the pernicious routine of the old school, have actually been most conducive to the successful cure. But if the patient dies, as is often the case, they quiet the sorrows of the mourning relatives by reminding them "that they had witnessed themselves that everything possible had been done for the now departed patient." Who would honor this careless and pernicious class with the name of *homœopathic physicians* after the laborious and salutary art? May their just reward await them, that, if ever sick, they may be cured after their own fashion!

[102] § 153. By arranging the characteristic symptoms, particularly of antipsoric medicines, Dr. von Bœnninghausen has lately merited our renewed gratitude by his significant little book: *Synopsis of the Sphere of the Main Effects of the Antipsoric Medicines* (*Uebersicht der Hauptwirkungs-Sphäre der Antips. Arz.*), Munster, by Coppenrath, 1833, and an Appendix to the same (comprising also, antisyphilitic and antisycotic medicines), attached to the second edition of his *Systematic Alphabetical Repertory of Antipsoric Medicines*, by Coppenrath, in Munster.

[103] § 160. This elevation of drug-symptoms above the analogous disease-symptoms, resembling an aggravation, has also been noticed by other physicians, whenever chance has placed a homœopathic remedy in their hands. When a patient, afflicted with the itch, complains of an increase of the eruption after having taken sulphur, the physician, ignorant of the real cause, comforts him with the assurance that more of the itch ought to come out before it can be cured; but he does not

know that it is a sulphur-eruption assuming the appearance of increased itch.

Leroy, *Heilk. für Mütter*, p. 406, says: "The eruption on the face cured by *Viola tricolor*, was at first aggravated by this medicine (Pansy or Heartsease)," but he does not know that this apparent aggravation was produced by the overdose of this medicine, which is in some respects homœopathic to the case. Lysons (*Med. Transact.*, vol. ii, London, 1772), says: "Elm bark is most sure to cure those cutaneous eruptions, which are increased in the beginning of its use." Had he administered this bark in very small doses, as he should have done in accordance with the similitude of symptoms, *i. e.*, in its homœopathic use, instead of giving it in enormous doses (common in allopathic practice), he would have accomplished a cure without, or at least, almost without this apparent intensification of the disease (homœopathic aggravation).

[104] § 161. Although the effect of medicines, the duration of which is naturally a long one, rapidly comes to a close in acute diseases, and most rapidly in the most acute diseases, this effect is, nevertheless, very enduring in chronic diseases (engendered by psora); hence antipsoric medicines frequently do not manifest such homœopathic aggravation in the first hours, but they produce it later, at various periods, during the first eight or ten days.

[105] § 181. The symptoms proceed from the remedy unless they were caused by a grave error in diet, a violent passion, a tumultuous process within the organism, the appearance or decline of the menses, conception, parturition, etc.

[106] § 183. Where the patient finds himself in a very distressed condition, notwithstanding the indistinctness of his symptoms (which rarely happens in chronic, but more frequently in acute diseases), a condition to be ascribed to the benumbed state of the nerves, which prevents the pains and complaints of the patient from being distinctly perceived, here opium will remove this depression of inner nervous sensibility, and the symptoms of the disease will become distinctly perceptible in the after-effect.

[107] § 188. One of the many pernicious theories of the old school.

[108] § 194. For instance, Aconitum, Rhus radicans, Belladonna, Mercurius, etc.

[109] § 197. Fresh itch eruption, chancre, sycotic excrescences.

[110] § 199. The remedies for sycotic disease, and the antipsoric remedies were unknown before my time.

[111] § 201. The fontanels of the old-school physician have a similar effect, in the form of artificial ulcers upon external parts; they soothe internal chronic complaints, but only for a very short time, and without curing them; on the contrary, they weaken and ruin the entire state of health, much more than the instinctive vital force could do by most of its metastases.

[112] § 203. Whatever internal medicines were used in the case, they only served to augment the disease, because these remedies possessed no specific curative power over the totality of the evil, but rather undermined the organism by weakening it, and by engrafting other chronic diseases upon it.

[113] § 205. Hence, for instance, I cannot recommend the use of the cosmic remedy, Arsenic, for the extermination of the so-called cancer of the lips or face (a product of highly developed psora ?), not only because this remedy is very painful and often unsuccessful, but more particularly because the fundamental disease is not in the least diminished by it, even if this dynamic remedy relieves that part of the body which is affected by a malignant ulcer; owing to this failure, the maintaining power of life is compelled to transfer the focus of the great inner disease to a more vital part (which is the case in every metaptosis), and to produce blindness, deafness, insanity, suffocative asthma, anasarca, apoplexy, etc. But this dubious local relief, effected in part by the removal of a malignant ulcer by the topical application of Arsenic, will, after all, succeed only where the ulcer has not attained a large size, and only while the vital force retains its energy; but during this same state of things, it is still possible to effect a complete cure of the original disease.

The same result may be observed after excision of cancer of the face or breast, and after enucleation of the encysted tumors; this is followed by more serious consequences, at all events, death is hastened; and notwithstanding the frequency of such a termination, the old school blindly pursues the same course in every new case, causing equally deplorable disasters.

[114] § 205. Itch eruption, chancre (bubo), condyloid excrescences.

[115] § 206. In making inquiries of this kind, we should not allow ourselves to be deceived by the assertions of patients or their attendants, who frequently state the cause of inveterate, nay, of the greatest and most protracted diseases, to be a cold taken many years ago (from wet, or cold drafts after being heated), or some previous fright, strain, or mortification (and even witchcraft), etc. Such causes are much too slight to produce an inveterate disease in a healthy body, to sustain it for years, and to augment it from year to year after the manner of chronic

diseases, produced by developed psora. Incomparably greater causes than those within the patient's recollection, must lie at the root of the beginning and progress of any significant and obstinate malady; those presumptive incidents can only serve as accessory causes, by which a chronic miasm is aroused.

[116] § 210. In painful diseases, for instance, of several years' standing, we frequently meet with gentle dispositions, commanding respect and compassion on the part of the physician for the patient. But as soon as the disease is conquered, and the patient restored to health—a possibility of frequent occurrence under homœopathic treatment—the physician will often be amazed and shocked at the frightful changes in the disposition of the patient. Ingratitude, obduracy, refined malice, and the most disgraceful and revolting caprices are then often seen to reappear, all of which were peculiar to the patient in times of health.

Persons who are patient in health, are often found in sickness to be obstinate, violent, and hasty, or intolerant and wilful, impatient or despairing; those who were previously chaste and modest, are then found lascivious and shameless. A bright intellect is not infrequently found to be dull; a person commonly of weak mind, on the other hand, will be more shrewd and sensible; while one of sluggish intellect, sometimes shows great presence of mind, and promptness, resolution, etc.

[117] § 213. Thus, Aconitum napellus will rarely or *never* produce a rapid or permanent cure in a patient of calm and complacent disposition, as little as Nux vomica will affect a mild phlegmatic, or Pulsatilla a happy, cheerful, and obstinate temperament; or as little as Ignatia proves efficacious in an unchangeable state of mind, inclined neither to fright nor to grief.

[118] § 222. Cases rarely occur, where a protracted disease of the mind or temperament subsides of its own accord (by the return of the inner disease into the coarser bodily organs). These are the rare cases in which an inmate of the lunatic asylum is dismissed seemingly cured. But for these instances, all mad-houses would remain filled to the roof, so that the multitude of candidates waiting for admission, could scarcely ever be accommodated in these institutions, unless vacancies were created by the death of some of the patients. *None are ever really and permanently cured in these establishments.* A strong proof, among many others, of the total inefficiency of the old practice, which allopathic ostentation ridiculously honors by the appellation of *rational practice.* How often, on the contrary, has not the true healing art, pure homœopathy, restored to these sufferers the possession of their mental and bodily health, returning them to their friends and to the world.

[119] § 224. It seems as if the mind received the truth of these rational admonitions with displeasure and sadness, and as if it acted upon the body for the purpose of restoring the disturbed equilibrium; but it appears also, as if the body, by means of its disease, reacted upon the organs of the mind and temperament, thus creating in them a higher state of excitement by again transferring its suffering to these organs.

[120] § 228. We behold with amazement, the hard-heartedness and recklessness of physicians of numerous establishments for the insane, not only in England, but also in Germany. Ignorant of the true manner of treating such diseases by means of effective homœopathic (antipsoric) *medicines*, these men content themselves with tormenting the poor sufferers, by the most violent blows and other tortures. By these unprincipled and revolting measures they degrade themselves beneath the rank of overseers of houses of correction; for the latter merely fulfil their duty in punishing offenders, while the former seem to vent their rage on the apparent incurability of mental diseases. In the abject consciousness of their professional inability, too ignorant to relieve, and too indolent to accept a more appropriate method of treatment, they maltreat those miserable but innocent sufferers.

[121] § 232. Two or three kinds of conditions (states or stages), may appear alternately. In double alternate conditions, for instance, certain pains may invariably appear in the feet, etc., as soon as a certain form of ophthalmia vanishes; which will again supervene, as soon as the pain in the limbs has temporarily disappeared. Convulsions and cramps may alternate directly with another affection of the body, or one of its parts. In threefold alternate stages of some constitutional (alltägigen) illness, periods of apparently improved health and of heightened mental and bodily powers (exaggerated hilarity, increased vivacity of the body and flow of spirits, unnatural appetite, etc.), may rapidly take place; whereupon sullenness and gloominess of temper, or an intolerable hypochondriac state of the mind, combined with various functional disturbances in regard to sleep, digestion, etc., may appear quite as unexpectedly; this, in its turn, may be replaced with equal suddenness by the moderate indisposition of ordinary times. The same is observable in many kinds of alternate conditions. Frequently not a trace is left of the previous stage, when the new one appears. In other cases only a few marks of the preceding alternate state are found when the new one appears. Little is left of the symptoms of the former condition, at the appearance and during the progress of the next. Sometimes the morbid alternate conditions are essentially of an opposite nature, *e. g.*, melancholy alternating periodically with hilarious insanity, or raving madness.

[122] § 235. Pathology, which is yet in its infancy, knows only of one intermittent (alternating) fever, also called ague (cold fever). This science assumes that there is no other difference than that of the time of recurrence of these attacks, which are accordingly styled quotidian, tertian, quartan, etc. But besides the periods of recurrence of intermittent fevers, there are differences of far greater importance. There are countless forms of such fevers, many of which cannot even be termed fever and ague, because their paroxysms consist only of heat; others have only a cold stage, with or without subsequent perspiration; still others, which are marked by coldness of the whole body, together with a sensation of heat, or by external heat with chills; others again, where one paroxysm consists only of rigors or coldness, with subsequent feeling of relief, but where the next paroxysm consists only of heat, with or without subsequent perspiration; others again, where the heat appears first and the chill afterwards; others again, where chills and heat are followed by apyrexia, and whereupon perspiration appears alone, constituting the second attack, often following many hours afterwards; others again, where perspiration is wanting altogether, or where the entire attack, without either chills or heat, consists only of perspiration, or where the perspiration is present only during the hot stage. Of this kind there are still innumerable other differences, particularly in regard to the collateral symptoms, such as the particular kind of headache, bad taste in the mouth, nausea, vomiting, diarrhœa, the absence or presence of thirst, the particular kinds of pain of the body or limbs, sleep, delirium, mental affections, convulsions, etc., occurring before, during, or after the chill; before, during, or after the heat; before, during, or after the perspiration, and countless other deviations of this kind. All of these are evidently intermittent fevers of very different kinds, each of which naturally demands its own (homœopathic) treatment. It must be confessed that almost all of them can be suppressed (as often is the case) by large and enormous doses of Cinchona bark, or its pharmaceutical preparation, sulphate of quinine; that is to say, their periodical recurrence (the type) is extinguished by this drug, though frequently not without increased and oft-repeated doses, but patients who had suffered from such intermittents unsuited for Cinchona, like all those epidemic intermittents traversing entire countries, and even mountains, are never cured by the mere extinction of their typical character. On the contrary, those patients only remain diseased in another way, and often much more seriously than before, by peculiar chronic Cinchona diseases, which resist even the efforts of the true healing art, though persisted in for a long time. Can such results be called *cures?*

[123] § 235. Dr. Von Bœnninghausen, who has done more in behalf of our salutary art than any other of my disciples, was the first to

furnish an admirable illustration of this subject, and he has facilitated the selection of appropriate remedies for the greatest variety of fever epidemics by his book, *Versuch einer Homœopathischen Therapie der Wechselfieber* (*An Attempt at Homœopathic Therapeutics of Intermittent Fevers*), 1833. Münster near Regensburg.

[124] § 236. This is illustrated by the not infrequent cases of death where a moderate dose of opium, administered during the cold stage of the fever, speedily destroyed life.

[125] § 244. Larger and oft-repeated doses of Peruvian bark, or even concentrated preparations of bark, like sulphate of quinine, may indeed rid such patients of the typical attacks of marsh-intermittents; but those who were deceived in this respect will remain diseased in another manner, unless relieved by antipsoric remedies.

[126] § 246. In the former editions of the *Organon* I have recommended that a single dose of a well-selected homœopathic remedy should be allowed to terminate its operation before the same or a new remedy is repeated, a doctrine derived from the certain experience that the greatest amount of good can scarcely ever be accomplished, particularly in chronic diseases, by a large dose of medicine (a retrogressive measure recently proposed), however well-selected; or, what amounts to the same thing, by several small doses administered in rapid succession, because a procedure of this kind will not permit the vital force to undergo imperceptibly the change from the natural disease to the similar drug-disease. On the contrary, it is usually excited to violent revulsive action by one large dose, or by the quick succession of several smaller doses, so that the reaction of the vital force, in most cases, is anything but beneficial, doing more harm than good. Therefore, while it was impossible to discover a more salutary method than the one proposed by me, it was necessary to obey the philanthropic rule of precaution, *si non juvat, modo ne noceat;* in accordance with which maxim the homœopathic physician, considering human welfare to be his highest aim, was to administer but one most minute dose at a time of a carefully selected medicine in a case of disease, to allow this dose to act upon the patient, and to terminate its action. I say *most minute*, since it holds good, and will continue to hold good as an incontrovertible homœopathic rule of cure, that the best dose of the correctly selected medicine will always be the smallest in one of the high potencies (X) for chronic as well as for acute diseases,—a truth which is the invaluable property of pure homœopathy, and which will continue to stand as an imperishable barrier to shield true homœopathy from quackery (Afterkünste) as long as allopathy (and no less the practice of the modern mongrel sect composed of a mixture of allopathy and homœopathy) continues like a

cancer to undermine the life of suffering men, and to destroy them by large doses of medicine.

On the other hand, practice proves to us that a single small dose may be sufficient, particularly in light cases of disease, to accomplish nearly all that could, for the present, be expected from the medicine, especially in the case of infants and very tender, susceptible adults. It also becomes evident that in many, nay, in most cases of very protracted and inveterate diseases (often aggravated by previous inappropriate drugs), as well as in serious acute affections, such a minute dose, even of our highly rarefied medicines, will be insufficient to produce all the curative effects that might, in general, be expected to result from the medicine. Hence it may undoubtedly be found necessary to administer several doses of the same medicine for the purpose of altering pathogenetically the vital force to such an extent, and to raise its curative reaction to such a degree of tension, as to enable it to extinguish completely an entire portion of the original disease, as far as this object could be reached by any well-selected homœopathic remedy. The best-selected medicine, in a single small dose, would perhaps bring some relief in such cases, but far from enough.

A careful homœopathic physician would scarcely dare to repeat the dose of the same remedy again and again, since no advantage was ever gained by such a course, but, on accurate observation, certain disadvantages have most frequently been seen to follow. Exacerbations have been commonly noticed, even after the smallest dose of the most appropriate remedy, whenever it was repeated for two or three successive days.

A homœopathic physician, convinced of the homœopathic fitness of his chosen remedy, and desirous of relieving his patient in a shorter time than he had hitherto succeeded in doing by means of a single small dose, naturally arrives at the conclusion that, as long as a single dose is to be administered (for reasons detailed above), this dose might as well be increased; and that instead of a single fine pellet moistened with the highest attenuation, six, seven or eight pellets, or even whole drops of the dilution might be given at once. But unexceptionally the result was less favorable than it should have been; often it was actually injurious and detrimental—an evil difficult to repair in a patient treated in that manner.

Neither will low potencies of the remedy, in large doses, lead to a better result.

Experience teaches that the desired object will never be gained by increasing the single doses of a homœopathic medicine for the purpose of raising the pathogenetic excitement of the vital force up to the point of sufficient curative action. The vital force would be too violently and too suddenly affected and aroused, than that it could have time to prepare for a gradual, even, and salutary counteraction; hence it endeavors to throw off the surplus of the medicinal assailant by vomiting, diarrhœa, fever, perspiration, etc. Thus the object of the inconsiderate physician is, in a great measure, placed out of reach, or entirely frustrated. Little or nothing is accomplished toward the cure of the disease; on the contrary, the patient is visibly weakened, and for a long time a repetition, even of the smallest dose of the same remedy, is not to be thought of, lest it should have an undesirable effect upon the patient.

A number of small doses, repeated for the same purpose in quick succession, will accumulate in the organism till they constitute, as it were, one large dose, and will produce the same evil result, except in some rare instances. The vital force, unable to recover during the interval even between small doses, is overtasked and overpowered, incapacitated to begin curative reaction, and compelled to continue passively the predominant drug-disease forced upon it. This process is similar to that produced by the large and accumulating allopathic doses of a drug, resulting in protracted injury to the patient, an event we are daily called upon to witness.

Now, in order to avoid the errors here pointed out, to gain the desired object with greater certainty than before, and to administer the selected remedy in such a manner that it may do the greatest amount of good to the patient without injury, and finally, in order that, in a given disease, the medicine may accomplish as much as could possibly be expected, I have recently adopted a peculiar course.

I perceived that, in order to pursue the correct medium course, we should be guided by the nature of the different medicines, as well as by the bodily constitution of the patient, and the magnitude of his disease. Let us take, for example, the use of *Sulphur* in chronic (psoric) diseases; its finest dose (*Tinct. Sulph.* X°), even in the case of robust persons afflicted with developed psora, is rarely to be repeated with advantage oftener than once in seven days; this space of time must be extended still more in the treatment of weakly and susceptible patients, when it will be well to administer such a dose only once in nine, twelve or fourteen days, to be repeated until the medicine ceases to be serviceable. In such cases it will be found that in psoric diseases rarely less than four, but often six, eight, and even ten such doses (*Tinct. Sulph.* X°), administered successively at such intervals, are required for the complete extinction of that portion of the chronic disease which Sulphur (to continue the example) is capable of extinguishing, provided no allopathic abuse of Sulphur had occurred previously. *In this manner, a newly originated (primary) itch-eruption attacking a sufficiently robust person, and even if it had extended over the whole body, can be cured in ten or twelve weeks by administering every seventh day a dose of tinct. Sulf.* X° (that is, with ten or twelve globules); nor will it often be necessary to make use of a few doses of Carbo veg. X° (also at the rate of one dose a week); the cure may, therefore, be perfected without the least external treatment, excepting frequent change of linen and well-regulated regimen.

Although from eight to ten doses of Tinct. Sulph. X° may be generally considered as sufficient in other great chronic diseases, it is, nevertheless preferable, instead of applying the doses in uninterrupted succession, to give a dose of another medicine which, next to Sulphur, is most homœopathic to the case (generally *Hep. sulph.*), after each, or after every *second* or *third* dose of the latter; and to allow this new dose to operate from eight to fourteen days before a second series of three doses of Sulphur is again resorted to.

Not infrequently the vital force is indisposed to submit to the action of several successive doses of Sulphur, even at the stated intervals, and however well the medicine may have been adapted to the chronic evil, the repugnance of the vital power will be indicated by some moderate sulphur-symptoms, which appear during the treatment. In this case it is sometimes advisable to give a small dose of Nux vom. X°, and to permit this to act from eight to ten days, so that nature may again become disposed to allow Sulphur in continued doses, to act quietly and with beneficial result. In some cases, Pulsatilla X° is to be preferred.

If Sulphur had been allopathically misapplied (even several years before), the vital force will resist the effects of that medicine, though decidedly indicated; in that case even, visible aggravations of the chronic disease will be manifested by the vital force, after the smallest dose of Sulphur, nay even after smelling of a pellet moistened with Tinct. Sulph. X. This is a deplorable circumstance, which renders the best medical treatment almost useless; and still it is only one out of numerous instances of allopathically maltreated chronic diseases, for which, however, we possess some means of reparation.

In such cases, it is merely necessary to let the patient apply one pellet moistened with Mercur. Metall. X to his nostrils, and to take a deep inspiration through the nose (stark riechen lassen), and to let this dose, applied through olfaction, operate for nine days, in order to make the vital force again susceptible of the beneficial effects of Sulphur (at least by smelling of Tinct. Sulph. X°, a discovery for which we are indebted to Dr. Griesselich of Carlsruhe).

Of the other antipsoric remedies (perhaps excepting *Phosph.* X) fewer doses are to be given at similar intervals (*Sepia* and *Silicea* are to be given at longer intervals, where they are homœopathically indicated, without intercurrent remedies), in order to extinguish all that the indicated remedy is capable of curing. *Hepar sulph. calc.* is rarely to be administered internally or by olfaction, in shorter periods than fourteen or fifteen days.

As a matter of course, the physician should be fully convinced of the accuracy of his selection of the remedy before attempting a repetition of doses.

In acute diseases, the time for the repetition of the proper remedy is regulated by the rate at which the disease runs its course; here it may often be necessary to repeat the medicine in twenty-four, sixteen, twelve, eight, four hours, and less, while the medicine, without originating new complaints, continues to produce uninterrupted improvement; but where this improvement is not sufficiently marked, considering the dangerous rapidity of the acute disease, the interval must be still further lessened. Thus in cases of cholera, the most rapidly fatal disease known to us, it is necessary in the beginning to give one or two drops of a weak solution of Camphor every five minutes, in order to insure speedy and certain relief; while in the more developed stages, we may be called upon to employ doses of Cuprum, Veratrum, Phosphorus, etc. (X°), every two or three hours; or to give Arsenicum, Carbo veg., etc., at similar intervals.

In the treatment of so-called nervous fevers and other continued fevers, the repetition of the dose of the effective medicine is also governed by the foregoing rules.

In pure syphilitic diseases, I have commonly found one dose of metallic Mercury (X°) to be sufficient. But not infrequently, two or three doses, administered at intervals of six or eight days, were necessary, whenever the least complication with psora was visible.

In cases where one remedy or another was strongly indicated, but where the patient is very excitable and weak, the application of a remedy by olfaction is more efficacious and safe than the administration of a substantial dose of homœopathic medicine, however fine and highly potentiated. This is done by holding the mouth of the vial, containing one small globule moistened with the medicine, first to one nostril, and if the dose is to be still more efficacious, also to the other nostril of the patient, who takes a momentary inspiration, the effect of which continues quite as long as that of the substantial doses; hence this process of olfaction is not to be repeated at shorter intervals, than if the medicine had been given in substantial form.

[127] § 249. Since experience proves that a dose of a specific homœopathic medicine can scarcely be prepared too small to produce a distinct improvement in a disease to which it is adapted (§§ 161, 279), it would be contrary to our purpose, and hurtful to repeat the same medicine, or to increase the *dose* in the absence of an improvement, or whenever an aggravation, however slight, should make its appearance; in doing so, we would be guilty of following the method of the old school, and of acting under the delusion that the small quantity of medicine (too small a dose) could not be efficacious. *Every aggravation evinced by new symptoms*—provided no errors have been committed with

regard to physical and moral regimen—*only proves the unsuitableness of the medicine last administered* in the case of disease, *but it never is an indication of the weakness of the dose.*

[128] § 251. I have discussed this subject more fully in the introduction to Ignatia (*Mat. Med.*, Part 2d).

[129] § 253. The indications of improvement with regard to mind and temperament, are only to be observed soon after the exhibition of the medicine, provided the dose had been *sufficiently small* (*i. e.*, as small as possible); an unnecessarily large dose, even of the most homœopathically adapted medicine, acts too violently, disturbing the mind and temperament too much, and too continuously in the beginning, to allow the improvement in them to be seen *early*. I must remark here, that this necessary rule is most frequently violated by conceited beginners in homœopathy, and by those who come over from the ranks of the old school. Actuated by inveterate prejudices, they shun the smallest doses of the highest dilutions of medicines in these cases, and are, therefore, deprived of the great advantages and blessings derived from a method, which has been established as salutary by countless experiences; they cannot achieve as much as true homœopathy can accomplish, and hence, unjustly claim to be its disciples.

[130] § 259. The distant and mellow tones of the flute which, in the silent hours of night, would melt a tender heart, and call forth celestial emotions and religious sentiments, are drowned by the discordant and tumultuous sounds of the busy day.

[131] § 260. Coffee; Chinese tea, or other herb teas; beer containing medicinal vegetable substances unadapted to the condition of the patient; so-called cordials, prepared from medicinal spices; all kinds of punch; spiced chocolate; scented water and perfumes of various kinds; highly odorous flowers cultivated in the chamber; medicated tooth-powder or washes; perfumes inclosed in bags or cushions; highly seasoned food or sauces; spiced pastry or ices; raw medicinal herbs in soups; pot-herbs, tender shoots and roots possessing medicinal properties; old cheese and tainted animal food, or the flesh and fat of pigs, ducks, geese, or young veal, and acid food, etc., all of which produce collateral medicinal effects, are carefully to be kept from patients of this kind. Excesses at table; the excessive use of sugar and salt, as well as spirituous liquors; heated rooms; woollen clothes next to the skin (which, in warm weather, is first to be replaced by cotton and then by linen); sedentary habits in close apartments; passive exercise, such as riding, driving, rocking; protracted suckling of infants; the habit of sleeping in bed too long after dinner; nocturnal occupa-

tions; the enervating effects induced by the perusal of obscene books; objects of anger, grief, and vexation; the passion for gaming; excessive exertion of mind and body; residence in a marshy locality; damp rooms; penurious living, etc.: all these conditions and circumstances should be carefully avoided and removed, lest the cure might be impeded or rendered impossible. Some of my disciples appear to impose unnecessary restrictions on their patients, by prohibiting a still greater number of quite indifferent things, a course which is not to be sanctioned.

[132] § 263. This, however, is rare. In purely inflammatory diseases, for instance, where Aconite, a medicine easily counteracted in the organism by the use of vegetable acid, is indispensable, the patient generally experiences a desire for pure cold water.

[133] § 266. All crude animal and vegetable substances possess a greater or less amount of medicinal properties, and each, after its own manner, is capable of altering the sensorial condition (health) of man. Those plants and animals used as food by civilized nations, are preferable on account of the large amount of nutritious matter contained in them; they also differ from others in this, that the medicinal properties of their crude condition are less prominent, and that these properties are diminished by culinary processes; for instance, by pressing out the hurtful juices (like that of the South American Cassava), by fermentations (like that of rye flour when made into dough for bread; the preparation of sourkraut and pickles, without vinegar), by smoking, by heat (in boiling, frying, broiling, roasting, baking), by which means the medicinal elements are partially destroyed and evaporated. Through the addition of salt or vinegar (in pickling and preparation of sauces and salads), these animal and vegetable substances may lose a part of their medicinal properties, but injurious qualities of another kind are produced.

Plants, even, of strong medicinal properties are partly or wholly deprived of their strength by such modes of treatment. All roots of the iris species, horseradish, arum, and the peonies lose nearly all their medicinal strength by perfect desiccation. The juice of the most powerful plants is often transformed into an inert, pitchy mass by the ordinary temperature employed in the preparation of extracts. By being allowed to stand still for a long time, the expressed juice of deadly plants is often rendered inert; even at a moderate temperature it rapidly passes into vinous fermentation; being thus deprived of much strength, it grows sour, and finally putrid, whereby all its peculiar medicinal properties are destroyed. The amylaceous sediment, when purified, is perfectly harmless like ordinary starch. Even in the process of sweating, to which a closely packed mass of herbs would be exposed, a great portion of their medicinal properties are lost.

[134] § 267. Buchholz (*Taschenbuch für Scheidekunst u. Apoth.*, 1815, Weimar, I, VI) assures his readers, uncontradicted by his critic in the *Leipziger Literatur-Zeitung*, 1816, No. 82, that we were indebted for this excellent method of preparing medicines to the campaign in Russia, whence it was introduced into Germany. He conceals the fact that this discovery and its description had been made known by me two years before the Russian campaign, although he quotes my own words from the first edition of the *Organon of the Rational Healing Art*, § 230 (the *Organon* appeared in 1810), and the annexed note. Thus the origin of an invention is rather to be sought in the wilds of Asia than to attribute the honor to a German who justly claims it. Although alcohol was formerly sometimes mixed with vegetable juices to preserve them for the purpose of preparing extracts, it was never done with the intention of administering them in this form to patients.

[135] § 267. Although equal parts of alcohol and of fresh juice are the usual proportion effecting the subsidence of fibrous and albuminous matter, nevertheless a double quantity of alcohol is required for plants containing much viscid mucus, or an excess of albumen. Plants containing but little juice, like oleander, boxwood, yew tree, ledum, sabina, etc., should first be crushed into a fine pulp, and then stirred up with a double quantity of alcohol, so that the juice may combine with it, and being thus extracted by the alcohol it may be strained. These substances may also be dried, reduced to powder, ground with sugar of milk to the third trituration, and then farther diluted by potentiation after dissolving a grain of the trituration (cf. § 271).

[136] § 268. In order to preserve such substances in the form of powder, a precaution, hitherto not generally known to apothecaries, was requisite, in the absence of which these animal and vegetable substances, though perfectly dry, could not be kept in well-closed bottles. Crude, unpowdered vegetable substances, however dry, still contain a certain degree of moisture as a necessary condition for the cohesion of their structural particles. Although this moisture does not prevent the entire unpowdered drug from continuing in a dry state, it will nevertheless prove to be excessive for the preservation of a substance in a finely powdered state. Vegetable or animal substances, which are quite dry when whole, will, when finely pulverized, form a somewhat moist powder, which cannot be kept in closed vessels without being rapidly spoiled by mould unless previously freed from the excess of moisture. This is best done by spreading the powder in a shallow tin pan with a high rim, floating on boiling water (water-bath), and stir-

ring it till it has become so dry, that its small particles no longer adhere together in lumps, and until they can be separated and blown off like fine sand. In this state these fine powders may be preserved *forever* without deterioration in well-stoppered and sealed glasses, where they will retain their original and perfect medicinal strength *free from mould and mustiness.* The best plan is to protect the glasses from daylight in covered jars or boxes. Animal and vegetable substances, kept in glasses which are not perfectly air-tight, and kept from the access of sun and daylight, will in time lose more and more of their medicinal virtues even in their entire state, but more particularly in the form of powder.

[137] § 270. Desirous of employing a certain rule for the development of powers of fluid medicines, I have been led by manifold experiences and accurate observations to prefer two instead of repeated strokes of succussion for each vial, since the latter method tended to potentiate the medicines too highly. There are, nevertheless, homœopathists who carry about with them homœopathic medicines in fluid form, and who still insist that these medicines were not found to have been more highly potentiated, thereby disclosing a want of accurate observation. I dissolved one grain of soda in half an ounce (1 Loth.) of water mixed with a little alcohol contained in a vial, two-thirds of which it filled; after shaking this solution uninterruptedly for half an hour, it was equal in potentiation and efficacy to the thirtieth development of strength.

[138] § 271. This subject is fully explained in the preface to the medicines in the third edition of the second part of the *Materia Medica.*

[139] § 272. Some homœopathic physicians have tried the plan of administering two medicines at a time, or nearly so, in cases where one of the remedies seemed to be homœopathic to one portion of the symptoms of the disease, and where a second remedy appeared adapted to the other portion; but I must seriously warn my readers against such an attempt, which will never be necessary even if it should seem proper.

[140] § 274. Supposing the right homœopathic remedy to have been administered in a well-considered case of disease, it would be preposterous to order the patient to drink some other medicinal herb-tea, to apply herb-cushions, medicated fomentations, injections, salves or ointments; a sensible physician will leave such practice to irrational allopathic routine.

[141] § 276. The praise which has lately been bestowed by some homœopathic physicians upon the larger doses, arises partly from their selection of lower potencies, such as I was in the habit of using twenty

years ago for want of better knowledge, and partly from the circumstance that the medicines were not quite homœopathically selected.

[142] § 276. See note to § 246.

[143] § 280. Let these ordinary practitioners ask mathematicians to demonstrate the truth, that, although a substance be divided into ever so many parts, *some portion* of this substance, however minute, must still constitute each one of these parts; that the most inconceivably minute fractional particle never ceases to be *something* of the original substance, and hence, that it can never become nothing. Physical sciences will teach them that there are great forces (potencies) which are entirely imponderable, like heat, light, etc.; and that, consequently, these must be far lighter than the medicinal contents of the smallest homœopathic doses Let them determine, if they can, the weight of angry words causing a bilious fever, or the weight of afflicting news that can kill an affectionate mother when she hears of the death of an only son; let them touch for fifteen minutes a magnet capable of supporting a hundred pounds, and be convinced by painful sensations that even imponderable influences may produce the most violent medicinal effects upon the human body; let some weakling of that class allow a strong-willed mesmerist to touch the pit of his stomach lightly with the point of his thumb for a few minutes, and the intolerable sensations produced by this process will make him repent of having set limits to the activity of boundless nature.

If an allopathic physician, in trying the homœopathic method, cannot summon sufficient courage to use highly rarefied doses, he should ask himself what risk he would incur in using them? If only ponderables were real, and imponderables unreal, then one of these seemingly insignificant doses would, at worst, be without any effect whatever,—a result far more harmless than that following too large a dose of allopathic medicine. Why will such a physician consider his want of experience, combined with prejudices, as more competent than experience established by facts observed throughout many years? In addition to this, it must be remembered that the power of homœopathic medicine is augmented (potentiated) by friction and succussion at each successive division and comminution. This development of powers, unknown before my time, is so great, that in latter years convincing experience has led me to make use of two succussions after each dilution, where formerly I employed *ten*.

[144] § 284. Supposing one drop of a mixture containing $\frac{1}{10}$th of a grain of medicinal substance to have an effect = A, then one drop of a higher dilution, containing $\frac{1}{100}$th of a grain of medicinal substance, would have an effect about equal to $\frac{A}{2}$; if it contains $\frac{1}{10000}$th of a grain of

medicinal substance, it would have an effect equal to $\frac{A}{4}$; if it contains $\frac{1}{1000000000000}$th of a grain of medicine, its effect would be $= \frac{A}{8}$; and in this progression, the volume of the dose remaining the same, the quadratic (or perhaps more than quadratic) diminution of medicinal substance will always reduce the effect of the latter only by about *one-half.* I have very often seen one drop of the decillionfold dilution of Nux vom. produce almost exactly *half as great an effect* as one drop of the quintillionfold dilution, administered under the same circumstances, and to the same person.

[145] § 285. For this purpose it is best to use fine sugar-pellets of the size of poppy seeds; one of these pellets moistened with medicine, and introduced into the vehicle, constitutes a dose containing about $\frac{1}{300}$ th part of a dose; for three hundred of such pellets are sufficiently moistened by one drop of alcohol. By placing one of these pellets upon the tongue, and without swallowing some liquid afterwards, the dose is considerably lessened. But if there are reasons for administering the smallest dose, and if, at the same time, a speedy effect is to be produced upon a very sensitive patient, it will only be necessary to smell of the medicine once (see note to § 288).

[146] § 286. The healing and intoxicating effects of the simplest stimulants only, such as wine and alcohol, are diminished by dilution with a large quantity of water.

[147] § 287. By the word *intimately* I mean to say, that if a drop of medicinal fluid is shaken up *once* with one hundred drops of alcohol—that is to say, if the vial containing both, has been subjected to one vigorous downward stroke of the arm, while the vial is held in the hand, an exact mixture must have taken place; but that the mixture of both will be made far more intimate by two, three, ten or more such strokes; *i. e.*, the medicinal power will have become more highly potentiated, and the spirit of this medicine will have been unfolded and developed in a higher degree, and made far more penetrant in its effect upon the nerves. Now if these high dilutions are to serve the desirable purpose of diminishing the dose, and of reducing its effect upon the organism, it would be well not to shake each of the twenty or thirty vials more than twice, so that the medicinal force may be but moderately developed. It would also be proper not to extend the time of trituration too far in making dry powder-dilutions; *e. g.*, a grain of some crude medicinal substance, having been mixed with one hundred grains of sugar of milk, should be triturated vigorously only for an hour; a grain of this trituration, mixed with one hundred grains of sugar of milk ($\frac{1}{10000}$th dilution), should also be triturated for an hour, and the third dilution ($\frac{1}{1000000}$th), prepared by mixing a grain of the preceding trituration with one hundred grains of sugar of milk, should also be triturated for

one hour, whereby the medicine is brought to a state of dilution, possessing a moderate development of strength. The process of making these preparations is more fully described in the prefaces to the third edition of the second part of the *Materia Medica*, 1833.

[148] § 287. The higher the process of dilution, combined with potentiation (by means of two succussions), is carried, so much the more rapid and penetrant the effect of the preparation will appear in its influence upon the vital force, and in altering the sensorial condition. This process, however, does not lessen the efficacy of the preparation much, even if it is carried up to $\overline{XX}$, $\overline{L}$, $\overline{C}$, and still higher, instead of stopping, as usual, at $\overline{X}$, which is generally sufficient. These higher degrees seem to differ from the lower ones only in having an effect of shorter duration.

[149] § 288. Homœopathic remedies will act with the greatest certainty and efficacy, particularly by smelling or inhaling them in the form of vapor emanating continually from a dry pellet impregnated with a highly rarefied medicinal solution, and contained in a small vial. The homœopathic physician should apply the mouth of the vial first to one nostril of the patient, and request him to inhale the air from the vial; and if the dose is to be somewhat stronger, the vial should also be applied to the other nostril, the patient inhaling more or less vigorously, in proportion to the intended strength of the dose, whereupon the vial should be replaced, well corked, in his pocket-case to prevent abuse. *Hence the physician may dispense entirely with the services of an apothecary, if he chooses to do so.* Globules (of which ten, twenty or a hundred weigh a grain) moistened with the thirtieth potentiated dilution, and then dried, retain their full strength undiminished for at least eighteen or twenty years (as far as my experience reaches), even if the vial had been opened a thousand times, provided, however, it had been well protected from heat and sunlight. In case the patient's nostrils were obstructed by coryza or polypus, he should inhale through the mouth while holding the aperture of the vial between his lips. A certain result may be obtained in the case of infants by holding the vial close to their nostrils during sleep. The inhaled medicinal vapor comes into immediate contact with the nerves distributed over the parietes of the cavities, through which it passes, and thus stimulates the vital force into curative action in the mildest, but at the same time, in the most energetic manner. This is much superior to all other modes of administering medicines by the mouth. Every kind of internal chronic disease not entirely ruined by allopathy, as well as the most acute diseases that can be cured at all by homœopathy (what indeed cannot be cured by it, except surgical diseases requiring manual skill ? , are most surely and effectually cured by this process of olfaction. But of the

great number of patients who, for a year past, have sought my aid and that of my assistant, there is scarcely one whose chronic or acute disease we had not treated successfully alone by means of olfaction. During the latter half of this year I became convinced of the fact (which I would not have believed before), that by this process of olfaction the power of the medicine is exerted upon the patient, at least in the same degree of intensity, and, in fact, more quietly, though quite as long as that of a large dose of medicine administered by the mouth, and that, consequently, the process of olfaction is not to be repeated at shorter periods than if the medicine were given in material doses by the mouth.

[150] § 289. Even patients deprived of their sense of smell are influenced and cured in an equally perfect manner by inhaling medicinal vapor through the nose.

[151] § 292. Friction (inunction) seems to enhance the effect of medicines only inasmuch as friction *per se* renders the skin and the living fibre more susceptible, and capable of feeling the strength of the medicine, and of imparting this sensation of change in the sensorial condition to the entire organism. If the inner surface of the thigh has been well irritated by friction, mercurial ointment merely laid on will act quite as powerfully as if this ointment had been vigorously rubbed into the spot, according to the usual mode of "inunction," as it is called. It still remains doubtful whether the substance of the metal itself is made to penetrate to the interior of the body by means of this so-called process of inunction, or whether it is taken up by the absorbent vessels, or whether neither of the two effects occur. But homœopathy scarcely ever demands the inunction of any medicine, and least of all, the use of mercurial ointment for curative purposes.

APPENDIX.

I CONSIDER it necessary in this place to allude to *animal magnetism* or mesmerism (called so after Mesmer, its discoverer), differing in its nature from all other curative agents. This remedial power, the existence of which is often denied, is imparted to the patient by the touch of a well-disposed person, exercising the full strength of his will. It acts in part homœopathically, by exciting symptoms similar to those of the disease to be cured, and is applied for this purpose by means of a single pass or stroke of the hands held flatwise over the body, and carried, during moderate exertion of the will, from the crown to the tips of the toes;[1] this process is efficacious in uterine hæmorrhages, even when death is imminent. The application of mesmerism also serves to distribute the vital force equally through the organism, when it is abnormally active in some parts, and deficient in others; *e. g.*, in cases of rush of blood to the head, and sleepless, anxious restlessness of debilitated persons, etc., where it should also be applied by means of a single, but more powerful pass of the hands. It is also capable of imparting vital power, and of supplying deficiency of the latter directly to a single debilitated part, or to the entire organism. This object is not to be reached with the same degree of safety and certainty by any power, except that of mesmerism, which obviates the disturbances arising from other kinds of medical treatment. An effect of this kind is obtained in single parts of the body, by applying the hands or tips of the fingers, and by directing a strong effort of good will upon the part suffering from inveterate debility, where an internal chronic evil has established its local symptoms. Cases of this kind are, *e, g.*, chronic ulcers, amaurosis, paralysis of single limbs, etc.[2] Many sudden and apparent cures, performed in all ages by mesmerists endowed with great natural power, belong to this category. But the most remarkable instances of the communication of human power were witnessed in the resuscitation of persons who, after having lain in a state of apparent death for a long time, were acted upon by the powerful will of a well-disposed man in the prime of life and vigor.[3] History records several undoubted instances of this kind.

These methods of applying mesmeric power, depend upon an influx of vital force from one body into another; it is, therefore, called positive mesmerism.[4] But there is another manner of applying it, which produces a contrary effect to the former, and is, therefore, known as negative mesmerism. Of this kind, are the mesmeric strokes employed in awakening persons from a state of somnambulism, as well as all those manipulations known as "calming" and "ventilating." The safest and simplest means of discharging the excess of vital power accumulated in some portion of a vigorous organism, consist in the application of negative mesmerism by means of the right hand with its extended palm, held parallel to and about an inch from the body, and carried by a rapid motion from the crown of the head to the tips of the toes.[5] The more rapidly this motion is made, so much the more effective will be the discharge of vital force. In a case of apparent death, for instance, occurring in a female previously healthy,[6] whose menses were suddenly arrested at their commencement, by some violent emotional disturbance, the excess of vital force, probably accumulated in the præcordial region, is discharged and restored to its equilibrium throughout the organism, by means of a rapid negative stroke of the hand, which will be followed by immediate resuscitation.[7] A gentle and less rapid negative movement of the hand will also allay the great agitation, and anxious sleeplessness occasioned in very excitable persons, by a positive pass too powerfully applied.

EXPLANATORY NOTES

TO THE APPENDIX.

---

[1] It is equal to the smallest homœopathic dose, which, however, achieves wonders if applied under proper circumstances. Incompetent homœopathic physicians frequently overwhelm their patients, suffering from obstinate complaints, with a rapid succession of doses of various medicines; though homœopathically selected and administered in high potentiated dilutions, these produce such a degree of overexcitement, that life is placed in jeopardy, and that the least subsequent dose of medicine would inevitably prove fatal. In such cases the harmonious and equal distribution of the vital power, repose, sleep, and recovery, can only be brought about by a gentle mesmeric pass, repeatedly executed by the hand of a well-disposed person, to the affected part.

[2] Although this process of supplying a deficiency of vital power, repeated from time to time, can never accomplish a permanent cure, in cases where, as above stated, a general internal evil lies at the bottom of the chronic local disease; nevertheless, this positive mode of strengthening and sustaining the organism with vital power (which is no more a palliative than food or drink, in satisfying hunger and thirst), is a great adjuvant to homœopathic medicines in the actual treatment of the entire disease.

[3] Particularly if this power had been exercised by men, such as are rarely met with, and who, while endowed with a very benevolent disposition, possess but *a very slight degree of sexual desire*, which they can suppress easily, and in whom, therefore, the subtle vital forces ordinarily employed in the production of seminal fluid, are always present in abundance, and in readiness to be imparted to other persons through the medium of touch, applied under the exercise of a strong will. A number of powerful mesmerizers with whom I was acquainted all possessed these peculiarities.

[4] These remarks concerning the decided and undoubted curative power of positive mesmorism, are by no means intended to apply to that exaggeration of the same, often practiced upon patients of weak nerves, who, being subjected to such manipulations for hours every day, at length experience an enormous change of their entire being, called somnambulism; a state in

which a human being seems removed from the sensual world into the spirit-world—an extremely unnatural and dangerous condition, by which men have often dared to attempt the cure of chronic diseases.

[5] It is a well-known rule, that a person who is to be subjected to either positive or negative mesmerism, must not be clothed, even in part, with silk.

[6] For this reason, a negative pass, particularly if energetically executed, is very injurious to a person of low vitality, suffering from chronic debility.

[7] A robust country lad, ten years of age, during some slight indisposition, was mesmerized by a woman who passed the ends of her thumbs several times rapidly and energetically from the epigastrium along the ribs, whereupon the boy became deathly pale, losing both consciousness and power of motion, so that he could not be aroused in spite of the most strenuous efforts, and was supposed to be dead. I caused his elder brother to make a rapid negative pass from the crown of the head to the feet, which at once restored the patient to consciousness and health.

ALPHABETICAL INDEX

TO THE

INTRODUCTION AND TEXT.